IDEA Advocacy for Children
Who Are Deaf or Hard-of-Hearing

A Question and Answer Book
for Parents and Professionals

IDEA Advocacy for Children Who Are Deaf or Hard-of-Hearing

A Question and Answer Book for Parents and Professionals

Bonnie Poitras Tucker, J.D.
Professor of Law
College of Law
Arizona State University
Tempe, Arizona

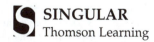
SINGULAR
Thomson Learning

Africa • Australia • Canada • Denmark • Japan • Mexico • New Zealand • Philippines
Puerto Rico • Singapore • Spain • United Kingdom • United States

NOTICE TO THE READER

COPYRIGHT © 1997 Delmar. Singular Publishing Group is an imprint of Delmar, a division of Thomson Learning. Thomson Learning™ is a trademark used herein under license.

Printed in the United States of America
4 5 6 7 8 XXX 03 02 01

For more information, contact Delmar, 3 Columbia Circle, PO Box 15015, Albany, NY 12212-0515; or find us on the World Wide Web at http://www.delmar.com

Library of Congress Cataloging-in-Publication Data:
Tucker, Bonnie Poitras, 1939-
    IDEA advocacy for children who are deaf or hard-of-hearing : a question & answer book for parents and professionals / Bonnie Poitras Tucker.
       p. cm. — (A Singluar audiology text)
    Includes index.
    ISBN 1-56593-896-8
    1. Children, Deaf—Education—United States. 2. Hearing impaired children—Education—United States. 3. Deaf—Government policy— United States. 4. Hearing impaired—Government policy—United States. I. Title. II. Series.
HV2537.T83 1997   97-23772
371.91'2'0973—dc21   CIP

Contents

Preface

This book is dedicated to parents of deaf and hard-of-hearing children everywhere. These parents are a special breed, facing choices and dilemmas unknown to other parents. And they are often forced to confront those choices and dilemmas while being bombarded from all sides with conflicting opinions and advice.

These parents have one thing in common: they want to do the best thing—to make the best choices—for their children. They deserve our admiration. They also deserve our full support and our respect. A big part of that support and respect is recognizing the right of parents to choose the type and form of education best suited to the needs of their individual children.

Parents of deaf and hard-of-hearing children face unique educational battles. Parents who want their children with hearing losses to be educated in mainstream classrooms must frequently fight school administrators who insist that those children must be educated in special schools for deaf children. Other parents who want their children with hearing losses to be educated in special schools for deaf children must sometimes fight school administrators who insist that those children must be educated in mainstream classrooms. Parents who want their children to be educated via the use of sign language must sometimes fight school administrators who insist the children must be taught oral/auditory communication. And parents who want their children to be educated via oral communication must fight school administrators who insist the children must use, and be taught, via sign language. For the most part, parents are left to fight these battles alone: one lone set of parents versus a comparative army of so-called educational experts.

This book is intended to assist parents in fighting those lonely educational battles. It outlines, in simple, understandable terms, the rights granted to deaf and hard-of-hearing children by the Individuals with Disabilities Education Act (IDEA), and addresses, in question and answer form, the most significant issues that parents of children with hearing losses must be aware of to assert those rights effectively on behalf of their children.

This book is written for ALL parents of children with hearing losses. In recognition of the ultimate right, and responsibility, of parents to make important choices for their children, this book offers guidance to assist parents in obtaining whatever educational benefits they deem necessary and appropriate for their deaf and hard-of-hearing children. In some contexts, therefore, the book addresses, in separate discussions, the most effective approaches for parents to utilize when negotiating or fighting for segregated education, integrated education, auditory or oral education, education via use of cued speech, or education via use of sign language for their children. In most contexts, however, the rights to be asserted and pursued on behalf of children with hearing losses are common to all such children. Those rights are discussed in generic terms.

At times this book may seem to take an adversarial position— to focus on legal action rather than on negotiation. This is because it is often when negotiation has failed—when parents and school districts are unable to reach a satisfactory resolution to differing opinions—that assistance is needed. Negotiation, however, is always preferred to legal action.

To parents of deaf and hard-of-hearing children everywhere: good luck. I hope that this book will serve to assist each of you in your sometimes lonely struggle to obtain educational services that are appropriate for your child, in light of his or her unique personal characteristics, your family situation, and your personal goals and objectives for your child.

But this book is not only for parents. It is also for professionals who assist parents in obtaining appropriate educational settings and services for their deaf and hard-of-hearing children. Professionals such as auditory/verbal specialists, audiologists, speech pathologists, sign language instructors, teachers, and parent advocates, all of whom routinely assist parents in devising appropriate educational programs for their deaf and hard-of-hearing children, often contact me and ask "where can I go to obtain an overview of what a deaf or hard-of-hearing child's rights are under the IDEA, so that I may better assist the child and his or her parents?" This book is intended to provide such professionals with the information they require. These professionals are to be commended for their hard work and dedication in assisting parents and their deaf and hard-of-hearing children. Hopefully, this book will aid in easing their struggles.

List of Acronyms

DOE	Department of Education (United States)
FAPE	Free and Appropriate Public Education
IDEA	Individuals With Disabilities Education Act
IEE	Independent Educational Evaluation
IEP	Individual Education Program
IFSP	Individual Family Service Program
LEA	Local Education Agency
LRE	Least Restrictive Environment
MDT	Multidisciplinary Team
OCR	Office of Civil Rights (of the Department of Education)
OSEP	Office of Special Education Programs (of the Department of Education)
SEA	State Education Agency
TTY	Teletypewriter Telephone for the Deaf (or Text Telephone for the Deaf)

CHAPTER 1

Introduction

This chapter briefly introduces the Individuals with Disabilities Education Act (IDEA) and the basic terminology used in that Act. Many of the topics mentioned in this introductory section will be discussed in greater detail later in this book.

Question: What is the IDEA?

Answer: In the 1970s it was found that state educational systems were not meeting the educational needs of children with disabilities. To help correct that problem, in 1975 Congress enacted the IDEA. The IDEA was originally known as the Education for All Handicapped Children Act or the Education of the Handicapped Act, and was commonly referred to as "public law 94-142." The IDEA is found at volume 20 of the United States Code, sections 1400–1485 [20 U.S.C. §§ 1400–1485]. The IDEA was amended in 1997 (The 1997 Amendments to the IDEA) to resolve areas of dispute and concern that have arisen since the Act's enactment in 1975.

Question: What are the purposes of the IDEA?

Answer: The IDEA has three primary purposes: First, to assure that all children with disabilities receive a *free, appropriate, pub-*

lic education that emphasizes special education and related services designed to meet their unique needs. Second, to protect the rights of children with disabilities and their parents or guardians. Third, to assist the states in providing for the effective education of all children with disabilities.

Question: Do all parts of the IDEA apply with respect to the rights of deaf and hard-of-hearing schoolchildren?

Answer: The IDEA contains eight subchapters, known as Parts A–H. Two parts are of primary concern to parents of deaf and hard-of-hearing schoolchildren: Subchapters II and VIII, known as Parts B and C (formerly Part H). Part B contains the "heart" of the IDEA—a set of procedural safeguards intended to protect the interests of children with disabilities from 3 to 21 years old. Part C authorizes states to receive grants from the federal government to develop and implement statewide systems to provide early intervention services for infants and toddlers (ages 0–3) with disabilities (including hearing losses). Only Parts B and C will be addressed in this book.

Question: The IDEA is a federal law. What must states do to comply with that federal law and what is the relationship between state and federal law with respect to the education of deaf and hard-of-hearing children?

Answer: The IDEA is basically a funding statute. The IDEA says that in order for a state to receive federal funds for its educational programs, the state must have an educational plan that incorporates the standards and procedures set forth in the IDEA. The state's educational plan must contain procedures to assure that children with disabilities are educated with children who are not disabled "to the maximum extent appropriate."

Since all states want to receive federal funds for their educational programs, all states have established plans to comply with the

IDEA. Although all states follow the basic premise of the IDEA, the individual state plans may contain some differing procedural requirements. A parent who is involved in a disagreement with educational administrators over his or her child's educational program will have to follow the procedures described in his or her state's plan. Generally, however, the most significant requirements are the same in all states, in accordance with the IDEA. Those requirements are explained in this book.

Question: **The IDEA requires that school districts provide children with disabilities with a "*free appropriate public education* which emphasizes *special education* and *related services* designed to meet their unique needs. . . ." What do those highlighted terms mean?**

Answer:

A. A "*free appropriate public education*," commonly called a FAPE, includes special education and/or related services provided at public expense that: (1) meet the standards of the State Educational Agency (SEA), and (2) are provided in accord with the Individualized Education Program (IEP) developed for a particular child with a disability. A student's school district, a part of the Local Education Agency (LEA), is responsible for providing that student with the FAPE described in the student's IEP. If the school district or LEA fails to do so, it becomes the responsibility of the SEA to step in and do so.

B. "*Special education*" means specially designed instruction to meet the unique needs of a child with a disability. Education is "special" under the IDEA because it is *both specially designed and meets the unique need* of the child.

C. "*Related services*" include support services that are designed to help a child with a disability to benefit from special education. Related services include transportation services, speech pathology, audiology services, physical therapy, occupational therapy, recreation (including therapeutic recreation and social work services), counseling (including rehabilitation counseling), psychological services, and medical services provided solely for diagnostic and evaluative purposes. Other services necessary to enable a child with a disability to benefit from special education services would also fall within this definition, such as transition services required to assist a student with a disability in making the transition from school to work or from high school to college or trade school.

Assistive technology devices and services, such as auditory trainers or frequency modulation (FM) systems, are also included in the IDEA. Although not specifically listed in the IDEA as part of the definition of special education or related services, assistive technology devices and services are required to be included in a child's IEP if they are necessary to provide the child with a free appropriate public education (FAPE).

Question: What is the "individualized educational program (IEP)"?

Answer: The IEP includes a document that is intended to be developed in a collaborative and cooperative effort between parents and school personnel. This document should precisely describe the child's abilities and needs, and set forth in detail the placement and services specially designed to meet those unique needs. The IEP is not only a document, however. It is the final step in a legally required process which must be followed for every child with a disability. Educators must work with parents, who are mandatory participants in this planning process, and who are provided with procedural safeguards in the event they disagree with the educators' plans. The IEP must be developed in accordance with detailed, legally required procedures.

Question: **A term that keeps popping up when the IDEA is mentioned is "least restrictive environment." What exactly does that term mean?**

Answer: Each child with a disability must be educated in the least restrictive environment (LRE) appropriate to meet his or her needs. The 1997 Amendments to the IDEA, as well as the regulations developed by the Department of Education (DOE) under the IDEA, provide that a child with a disability is to be removed from the regular educational environment only when "the nature or severity of the disability is such that education in regular classes with the use of supplementary aids and services cannot be achieved satisfactorily" [1997 Amendments to the IDEA; 34 Code of Federal Regulations § 300.550(b)(2)]. This LRE concept creates a presumption in favor of the integration of children with disabilities. When segregation can be avoided while still providing an appropriate education for a child with a disability, the IDEA requires integration with children who do not have disabilities.

The least restrictive environment concept is the heart of much controversy where deaf and hard-of-hearing children are at issue. This subject is discussed in great detail in chapter 4 of this book.

Question: **Does the IDEA apply to ALL children who are deaf or hard-of-hearing?**

Answer: No. The IDEA only applies to those deaf or hard-of-hearing children who require special education services, and are therefore classified as "educationally disabled." Some children with hearing losses do not require special education services, although they MAY require related services. Some children with hearing losses, for example, may be capable of being educated in regular, mainstream classes without any special educational programming or assistance, but they may require an amplification system (a related service) to enable them to hear what is said in the classroom.

A child who does not require special education services, and who is thus not classified as educationally disabled, is not entitled to receive related services at school expense under the IDEA, since if the child does not require special education services the IDEA does not apply. (The child may be entitled to such services under Section 504 of the Rehabilitation Act, however, as the answer to the next question explains.) The only exception to this rule regarding the inapplicability of the IDEA is when a state law specifically defines a particular related service, such as speech therapy or auditory training, as special education. If a state law defines speech therapy as special education, for example, and a child with a hearing loss is classified as educationally disabled because he or she requires speech therapy services, the child's school district would have to provide such speech therapy under the IDEA. Only rarely, however (if at all), will a state law label such services as special education services.

Question: **When a child with a hearing loss does *not* require special education services, and thus the IDEA does not apply, what can the child's parents do to obtain necessary related services, such as an FM system, for their child?**

Answer: The parents should request that the school district provide the necessary related services under Section 504 of the Rehabilitation Act. Section 504, which is found at volume 29 of the United States Code, section 794 [29 U.S.C. § 794], prohibits all recipients of federal financial assistance from discriminating on the basis of disability. Public school districts are recipients of federal financial assistance, and thus must comply with Section 504.

Under Section 504, school districts must provide children with disabilities with reasonable accommodations that will allow such children to receive nondiscriminatory educational services.

Thus, to comply with Section 504, school districts must provide a child with a hearing loss with related services necessary to allow the child to receive an appropriate education (such as an FM system) even if that child is not educationally disabled and not entitled to receive services under the IDEA. Section 504, like the IDEA, also requires that a child with a disability receive an appropriate education.

Parents frequently assume that if the IDEA does not apply to their child, the child is not entitled to necessary services at school expense. That assumption is incorrect. Public school districts must comply with Section 504 of the Rehabilitation Act, which is a very valuable law for deaf and hard-of-hearing children. Public school districts must also comply with Title II of the Americans with Disabilities Act, found at volume 42 of the United States Code, sections 12131–12165 (42 U.S.C. §§ 12131–65), which provides protections to school age children with hearing losses similar to those provided by Section 504.

CHAPTER 2

Development of an IEP

This chapter explains the concept and formulation of the Individual Education Program (IEP) that must be developed for every deaf and hard-of-hearing student who requires special education services to receive an appropriate education. Information is provided about the procedure to be followed when developing an IEP, the recommended substantive content of the IEP document, and the role that parents—and others—should play throughout this entire process. Means for obtaining appropriate evaluations of a child's strengths, weaknesses, and needs are outlined. Emphasis is placed on assisting parents to enable their children to meet appropriate goals, both during the particular school year at issue and in the future.

I. THE IEP MEETING

Question: **What must a school district do when a child who is deaf or hard-of-hearing and requires special education services enrolls in school?**

Answer: When a school district learns that a child in its district has a hearing loss and requires special education services, the school district must conduct a meeting within 30 days to develop an educational program for the child. This is known as an IEP meeting.

Question: **What if the child's hearing loss is unknown when the child is enrolled in school?**

Answer: Once a child is suspected of having a hearing loss, the school must refer the child to the school district's multidisciplinary team (MDT). The MDT is made up of school district personnel who are responsible for determining whether a child is disabled, and, if so, for developing the IEP, as discussed below.

If it is the child's parents who suspect the hearing loss, the parents should inform appropriate school authorities of their concern and request that the child be referred to the MDT.

Once a child is referred to the MDT (either because the school or the child's parents suspect a hearing loss), the school district must evaluate the child to determine if the child does have a hearing loss, and, if so, must determine whether the child requires special education services.

Prior to performing an initial evaluation of the child, however, the school district must obtain written consent from the child's parents. Pursuant to the 1997 Amendments to the IDEA, if the parents refuse consent for an evaluation, the school district may continue to pursue an evaluation by utilizing the mediation and due process procedures described in chapter 8 of this book.

Testing must be performed in the child's native language, and the tests must be specifically geared to assess specific areas of educational need. A general IQ test is not sufficient. A child with a hearing loss should be tested not only for the degree of his or her hearing loss, but for communication skills, social and emotional status, and academic status.

If it is determined that the child is in need of special education services, an IEP meeting must be conducted within 30 days.

If possible, the IEP should be developed before the school year begins so that it will be in effect when the school year starts. When a child is already receiving special education services in school this can be accomplished by developing an IEP for the coming year at the end of the previous school year. For some students, however, the LEA may need to meet and develop an IEP during the summer months to comply with the 30-day timeline. For others, when the child's disability and need for special education services is discovered in the midst of a school year, obviously the IEP will have to be developed in mid-year.

Question: What is the purpose of the IEP meeting?

Answer: The purpose of the IEP meeting is for the school district and the parents to jointly determine the needs of the particular child, and to develop an educational plan for the child that is appropriate to meet the child's needs.

Question: Who attends the IEP meeting?

Answer: At a minimum, the 1997 Amendments require that the following people must attend the IEP meeting:

1. The child's parents or guardians (unless they give up their right to attend);

2. a regular education teacher (if the child is participating or may participate in regular education);

3. a special education teacher or representative;

4. a representative of the education department who is qualified to supervise a specially designed education program for a child with a hearing loss, and who is knowledgeable about the general curriculum and about the school district's resources to assist children who are deaf or hard-

of-hearing (this person is known as the LEA representative and must be someone other than a teacher of the
child);

5. an individual who can interpret the instructional implica-
tions of evaluation results of the child (this person may also
be one of the teachers or the LEA representative mentioned
above).

Thus, there must be at least two, and probably three, different
representatives present from the educational system. If the child
has two teachers, a regular education teacher and a special education teacher, both teachers must attend. (Prior to the 1997
Amendments only one teacher was required to attend.)

In addition to the mandatory participants, other people may also
attend the IEP meeting:

If the child receives special assistance from a particular representative of the school district or local education agency, such as
a speech-language pathologist, that person should also be present at the IEP meeting. Personnel providing related services
should be included on the IEP team whenever particular related
services are to be discussed at the meeting.

In some cases, it is appropriate for the child to attend the meeting. Older children may want to be present at IEP meetings to
discuss plans for their educational programs. And, the IDEA
requires that the child be present when transition services are
being considered—to assist the student in making the transition
from school to work or from high school to postsecondary school.
Parents should have the child attend the IEP meeting whenever
it is felt that the child will understand the process and is capable
of presenting his or her thoughts or feelings.

When transition services are to be incorporated in the IEP, a representative from every agency likely to be responsible for provid-

ing or paying for transition services (such as the state department of vocational rehabilitation) must be invited to attend the IEP meeting.

Other individuals may also attend the IEP meeting at the discretion of the school district or the parents. Parents may bring anyone to the meeting who is familiar with either the education laws or the child's needs. For example, parents might wish to have an advocate or attorney present at the meeting. In some situations parents might wish to have a psychologist, speech and/or language therapist, auditory-verbal specialist, sign language teacher, or other expert who is familiar with their child's unique needs, present at the meeting. The school district may also invite such persons to attend the meeting.

Question: **Should parents have an advocate or attorney present at the IEP meeting?**

Answer: If there is any likelihood that the school district and the parents will be in disagreement over the IEP to be devised for the child, it is advisable for parents to have an advocate or attorney present at the meeting. Further, it is advisable for parents to have experts who know their child's abilities and needs attend the meeting. If parents do not invite such persons to the IEP meeting, the parents are likely to be outnumbered by representatives of the education department. Moreover, since representatives of the education department are speaking from the perspective of "experts," parents who are not education experts tend to be intimidated and are not always able to effectively present their ideas and concerns to those experts.

Question: **Can the school district be required to pay for an attorney to assist parents in an IEP meeting, at least when the parents and the school district are involved in a dispute over the IEP to be developed for a child and the attorney is successful in having the dispute resolved in favor of the parents?**

Answer: Pursuant to the 1997 Amendments to the IDEA, attorneys' fees may not be awarded with respect to IEP meetings unless: (a) the IEP meeting was conducted as a result of a due process hearing or court proceeding (explained in chapter 8 of this book), or (b) the state convenes a meeting for mediation purposes (again explained in chapter 8). The 1997 Amendments thus reverse some earlier case decisions allowing attorneys' fees to be recovered for IEP meetings.

Question: Suppose parents cannot afford an attorney. What alternative assistance is available?

Answer: Many states have state-funded legal service agencies that provide assistance to parents of children with disabilities, such as a "Center for Disability Law," or a similar state agency. Such agencies may provide the services of specially trained nonlawyer advocates, who are familiar with the IDEA and parents rights under that law, and who sometimes assist parents in IEP meetings. In many states, nonprofit community legal service organizations provide assistance to parents of children with disabilities, in the form of trained advocates, paralegals, or attorneys.

Parents who are unable to locate such agencies or organizations in their states may wish to contact the National Association of the Deaf (NAD) or the NAD Law Center in Silver Springs, Maryland, or the Alexander Graham Bell Association for the Deaf in Washington, D.C., and ask for appropriate referrals. In addition, parents may ask for referrals from state agencies or councils for the deaf or from state information and referral services. (Information is provided in the Appendix.)

Question: How often must an IEP meeting be held?

Answer: An IEP meeting must be held at least once a year to review and update or revise the child's IEP.

Question: **Can parents request an IEP meeting at other times?**

Answer: Yes. Both parents and the school district can request an IEP meeting at any time that either does not believe that a child's current IEP is appropriate. If parents request such a meeting, the school district/local education agency is responsible for setting up and conducting the meeting. The IDEA does not provide for a specific time by which such a meeting must be conducted, but, to meet the intent of the law, the meeting would have to be held within a reasonable time from the request.

Question: **What is the school district's responsibility with respect to scheduling the IEP meeting?**

Answer: The school district must notify parents sufficiently in advance of an IEP meeting to ensure that the parents will be able to attend. The notice must inform parents of the time, place, and purpose of the meeting, as well as who will be present at the meeting as representatives of the education department. The notice may be either oral or written, or both.

Question: **What if the parents cannot attend the meeting at the scheduled time?**

Answer: The IEP meeting must be scheduled at a time and place that is mutually agreeable to the parents and the school district. If parents are unable to attend a meeting scheduled by the education department, another meeting time must be arranged. A school district must make a good-faith effort to reach an agreement with parents regarding the scheduling of an IEP meeting. The school district, however, may also consider its own scheduling needs.

Question: **Can the school district hold an IEP meeting without the parents?**

Answer: Generally, NO. The only time a school district can hold an IEP meeting without the parents is when the school district has made several unsuccessful attempts to arrange a meeting at which the parents could be present, and when such unsuccessful attempts are documented.

There have been instances in which school personnel have held unofficial IEP meetings among themselves and sent the resulting IEP forms to a child's parents for the parents to sign. This is NOT permissible under the IDEA. If this happens, parents should request a formal IEP meeting, and ultimately, if necessary, a due process hearing (explained in chapter 8).

Question: If parents use sign language, or speak another language, such as Spanish, must the school district/local education agency provide an interpreter for the IEP meeting?

Answer: Yes. The school district must do whatever is necessary to ensure that the parents understand the proceedings at an IEP meeting, including arranging for a needed interpreter.

Question: May an IEP meeting be held via telephone?

Answer: Yes, if all parties agree. That is not recommended practice, however.

Question: May parents review their child's school records prior to the IEP meeting?

Answer: Yes. The IDEA specifically states that parents are entitled to inspect and review all school records relating to their child. The school district must explain and interpret the records if asked to do so by parents.

A school district may charge a fee for copying the records for the parents if the fee would not effectively prevent the parents from reviewing the records.

The school district must comply with the parents' request to review the records prior to the IEP meeting (and, if no IEP meeting is scheduled, the district may not take more than 45 days to comply with the parents' request).

If the parents believe that any information in those records is inaccurate or misleading, the parents can request that the records be amended. If the school refuses to amend the information, the parents have the right to a hearing conducted by the educational agency. If the parents succeed at the hearing, the records must be amended. If the parents do not succeed at the hearing, the parents may place a statement in the child's records commenting on the information that is alleged to be inaccurate or misleading.

Question: What should parents do to prepare for an IEP meeting?

Answer: Prior to the IEP meeting, the parents should carefully review their child's school records (if any exist), as explained in the answer to the previous question. Second, the parents should carefully review all evaluations conducted of their child. Parents are entitled to review all such evaluations, including test protocols. If the parents disagree with the findings, they should obtain an independent evaluation of their child, as explained in the answer to the next question.

Third, the parents should determine who will be attending the IEP meeting on behalf of the education department (the school district is required to provide parents with that information). If the parents feel that other school personnel should attend the meeting, they should request that the school district include those persons.

Fourth, the parents should make a list of their child's strengths, weaknesses, and needs—including the type of environment the child will require, the communication mode the child should use, and the services necessary to help their child learn. They should identify realistic goals for the child to achieve during the school year and prioritize those goals in order of importance. Basically, the parents should decide what they would like to see occur in their child's program.

In setting short-term goals, parents should consider their ulti-mate, long-term goals for their child. What do they envision for their child when the child reaches the age of 21? What kind of lifestyle do they hope their child will have as an adult? Parents should keep in mind that the decisions they make with respect to their child's early education will greatly influence the child's entire life. It is imperative that the short-term goals established for the parents further those ultimate long-term goals.

Fifth, the parents should consider who they wish to bring with them to the meeting (such as an advocate or attorney, educational or other experts) and invite such persons to attend the meeting.

Finally, the parents should prepare written notes to bring to the meeting that address their concerns, opinions, and expectations for their child and the delivery of educational and related services to their child. The parents should have a clear, concise plan for their child's education and should be prepared to present their ideas firmly but nicely. Parents should be cooperative and pleas-ant, but should not feel the need to defer to the opinions or deci-sions of school personnel.

Question: **When and how should parents obtain an indepen-dent educational evaluation of their child?**

Answer: Parents always have the right to have an independent educational evaluation (IEE) of their child. Parents should obtain such an IEE if for any reason they do not believe the school dis-trict's evaluation is appropriate or adequate.

If parents do not know where to obtain an IEE they may ask the school district for assistance, and the district must provide the parents with information explaining where an IEE may be obtained.

Question: Must school districts pay for the Independent Educational Evaluation (IEE)?

Answer: In some cases the school district/local education agency will be responsible for paying the cost of the IEE. If, however, the school district claims that the IEE is not necessary, because the school district's own evaluation is appropriate or because the IEE simply duplicates the evaluation performed by the school district (or by an outside entity on behalf of the school district), the school district is entitled to initiate a due process hearing on the issue of its responsibility for payment. If the school district succeeds at the due process hearing, it will not be required to pay for the IEE (unless the ruling of the hearing officer is overruled by a court).

Ultimately, the question of whether the school district must pay for the IEE is a complex issue that will be resolved on a case-by-case basis. Parents should be aware, however, that courts have held that parents are entitled to only one IEE at public expense, and that a school district is not responsible for paying for multiple evaluations that are duplicative or corroborative.

To maximize the likelihood that the school district will be required to pay for an IEE, parents should ensure that the IEE takes a different approach, or focuses on different issues, than the school district's evaluations. Parents should be prepared to explain why the school district's evaluations are inappropriate, and how and why the IEE is different.

Question: **Is there a time frame in which the school district must request a due process hearing on the issue of its responsibility for payment of an Independent Educational Evaluation (IEE)?**

Answer: The IDEA does not specify such a time frame. The Office of Special Education Programs (OSEP), however, has stated that the school district must do one of two things within a reasonable time: (a) pay for the IEE, or (b) request a hearing to show that its evaluation is appropriate.

Question: **What should the IEP team (the persons attending the IEP meeting) consider when devising the child's IEP?**

Answer: Pursuant to the 1997 Amendments, the IEP team must consider the child's strengths, the parents' concerns for enhancing the education of their child, and the results of the initial or most current evaluation of the child. The team should also consider the student's current school records (if the child is currently in school), the current IEP for the child (if one exists), any independent educational evaluations of the child, and any other relevant information. If the child is not currently in school the IEP team should also consider results of the child's evaluations and tests, information about programs the child has been attending or therapy the child has been receiving (if any) and the child's progress in such programs or therapy, information about the child's current communication mode and abilities, information about the family's communication preference, and any other relevant information.

If the child has behavioral problems that impede his or her learning or the learning of others, the 1997 Amendments require the IEP team to consider behavioral interventions, strategies, and supports to address those problems.

The 1997 Amendments also require the IEP team to consider whether the child requires assistive technology devices and services.

There are special considerations involved with respect to deaf or hard-of-hearing children, as noted in the question below.

Question: **What, if anything, must the IEP team consider with respect to the communication needs of deaf and hard-of-hearing children?**

Answer: The 1997 Amendments require the IEP team to consider a deaf or hard-of-hearing child's

> language and communication needs, opportunities for direct communications with peers and professional personnel in the child's language and communication mode, academic level, and full range of needs, including opportunities for direct instruction in the child's language and communication mode.

This provision is to be implemented in accord with the policy guidance entitled "Deaf Students Education Series," published in 1992 by the United States Department of Education [57 *Federal Register* 49274, October 30, 1992]. The Policy Guidance incorporates suggestions made in the Report of the Commission on the Education of the Deaf, which provides that an IEP for a child who is deaf or hard-of-hearing must consider the following:

1. The communication needs of the child;

2. the family's preferred communication mode;

3. the linguistic needs of the child;

4. the severity of the child's hearing loss and potential for using his or her residual hearing;

5. the child's academic level; and

6. the child's social, emotional, and cultural needs, including opportunities for peer interaction and communication.

On its face, this 1997 addition to the IDEA seems more geared to ensuring opportunities for deaf or hard-of-hearing children to be educated in sign language programs than in oral programs. It is important to note, however, that the Report of the Senate Committee on Labor and Human Resources with respect to the 1997 Amendments explains that the 1997 Amendments are intended to reinforce the longstanding policies of: (a) having children with disabilities be educated with children without disabilities to the maximum extent possible, and (b) providing a continuum of alternative placements for children with disabilities (which requires the availability of both sign language and oral programs).

It remains to be seen how school districts, hearing officers, and the courts will interpret the 1997 provision relating to the communication needs of children who are deaf or hard-of-hearing.

Question: What factors should the IEP team review?

Answer: If the child is currently in school, the IEP team should first determine whether the current IEP is adequately meeting the child's needs. Have current annual goals, including measurable benchmarks and short-term objectives, been satisfied? If not, those objectives and goals must be reevaluated, and new goals and objectives must be established. If annual goals and short-term objectives have been satisfied, the team should establish appropriate new goals and objectives. The team should also consider whether the child is ready to enter a program in a less restrictive environment.

If the child is not currently in school, the IEP team should consider all relevant information when devising an IEP for the child, as explained in the answer to the previous question.

Question: Whose rights or wishes take priority in the IEP process—those of parents or the school district?

Answer: Neither. Parents and school officials stand on equal footing in the IEP process; neither parents nor school officials have a greater say in the decision-making process.

Again, while cooperation is the goal, parents should be aware that they are NOT required to accept the school's proposed placement or services. It takes a lot of courage for parents to stand up to the so-called experts. But parents have the legal right to do just that. If parents are not happy with the services proposed by the school, or do not feel that suggested services are necessary or appropriate, they must be prepared to say so, and to "stick to their guns" without wavering or waffling.

But it is not enough for parents to object to the school district's proposed services. Rather, to have effective input into their child's educational program parents must be prepared to propose alternatives that are geared to meet the realistic goals they have established for their child.

Parents should attempt to work with school officials as cooperatively as possible, without forfeiting their own ideas, objectives, or goals for their child. Parents should listen to what school officials have to say, and recognize that the educators may also want to do the best thing for children with disabilities (but that they may feel constrained to do so due to increasing budget cuts and orders to tighten the belt). Ultimately, however, parents should remember that they stand on equal footing with school authorities with respect to the development of their child's IEP. Thus, parents should stick to their bottom line, and not permit educators to intimidate them.

Question: **What happens if school representatives and the child's parents are not able to reach a consensus with respect to the appropriate IEP to be developed for the child?**

Answer: In the event parents disagree with school officials, and the disagreement cannot be resolved between the two, the Multi-disciplinary Team (MDT) will determine what is to be stated in the IEP. Parents, however, are not required to sign an IEP they do not agree with, and, indeed, should refuse to sign such an IEP. At this point, either the parents or the school district may request a due process hearing, as explained in chapter 8.

Question: **Must the school district keep reports of the IEP meeting (and the IEP itself) confidential?**

Answer: Yes. Confidentiality is required.

Question: **May IEP meetings be recorded or videotaped?**

Answer: Yes. IEP meetings may be recorded or taped at the discretion of either the parents or the school district, with or without the consent of the other party. If the school district records or videotapes the meeting, however, it must keep the recordings or tapes confidential.

II. THE IEP DOCUMENT

Question: **What information should the IEP document contain?**

Answer: As amended in 1997, the IDEA requires that, at a minimum, the IEP statement must contain the following information:

1. The child's present educational performance levels.

2. The annual goals for the child, including short-term instructional objectives.

3. A statement of the special education, related services, and supplementary aids and services to be provided to or for the child.

4. An explanation of the extent, if any, to which the child will not participate with nondisabled children in the regular classroom.

5. A statement of any special modifications in student assessment procedures that the child may require.

6. The dates on which it is anticipated that the services listed will be initiated, and the expected frequency, location, and duration of those services.

7. Beginning at age 14, and every year thereafter, a statement of the child's needed transition services related to the child's course of study (to ensure that the child's educational program is planned to help the child reach his or her goals for life after secondary school).

8. If appropriate, beginning at age 16, a statement of needed transition services for the child, including a statement pertaining to the responsibilities of various agencies to provide such services.

9. A statement of how the child's progress toward annual goals will be measured, and how the child's parents will be regularly informed of the child's progress (such as by "IEP report cards"—a process by which schools will provide parents with regular report cards indicating the extent to which their children are making progress under their IEPs).

In addition, beginning at least one year before the child reaches the age of majority under state law (i.e., 18 or 21 as the state provides), the IEP must include a statement that the child has been informed of his or her rights under Part B of the IDEA.

Some states require that other criteria be listed in the IEP, but at a minimum the IEP must contain the above elements. Parents should, however, be aware of the requirements specified in their state law.

Question: **What should parents emphasize when helping to develop an IEP for their child?**

Answer: Parents should ensure that the IEP devised for their child is as detailed and specific as possible and addresses the entire scope of the child's educational experience. For example:

If a child is to receive speech therapy, the IEP should list the number of hours per week the child will see the therapist, how long the therapy sessions will last, who will provide the therapy, whether the sessions will be individual or group sessions, and what the specific short-term and long-term goals for the child are. (A short-term goal might, for example, be for the child to learn to pronounce the sounds "L," "R," and "S" properly, while the long-term goal might be for the child to improve general speech intelligibility. A short-term goal might be for the child to speak in three-word phrases, while the long-term goal might be for the child to speak in full sentences.)

If the child is to receive sign language instruction, the IEP should list similar factors. Further, the IEP should identify the specific signing system or systems to be utilized (i.e., signed English, American Sign Language, etc.) And, if it is determined that, to enhance the child's overall educational experience, it is necessary for the child's parents to receive sign language instruction, the IEP should specifically incorporate that factor and should specify the same detailed information.

For most children who are deaf or hard-of-hearing, particularly in the early years, language development is of primary concern. The IEP should clearly address, in a series of "stepping stones" or short-term goals, what steps will be taken to improve the language level of the child, and what the expected outcome is at the end of the year. The annual goal should be set at the highest level that the child has a reasonable chance of attaining during the school year. Care should be taken, however, not to underestimate the abilities or capabilities of children with hearing losses.

If the child needs to develop his or her social skills, as many deaf and hard-of-hearing children do, that factor should be listed in the IEP, and the IEP should state specifically what methods are to be utilized in assisting the child to develop such skills. In the early grades, for example, the teacher might implement a "buddy" system, form "play groups," and/or organize group play at recess and lunchtime. In later grades extracurricular activities may be appropriate.

If it is deemed appropriate for the child to participate in extracurricular activities, those activities should be specified in the IEP. This is particularly important for older children in mainstream programs which have "no pass, no fail" rules, pursuant to which a child who does not pass all of his or her classes or maintain a certain grade point average is prohibited from participating in extracurricular activities. If participation in extracurricular activities is specified in the child's IEP, such a rule will not apply to prevent the child from participating in the specified activities. This may be crucial for children who are deaf or hard-of-hearing, who may benefit substantially from participating in extracurricular activities, and who might be unduly penalized by a rule requiring a specified grade point average as a prerequisite to such participation.

Parents may also want the IEP to address the issue of discipline. If the child has behavior problems relating to his or her hearing loss, the IEP should address the manner in which those problems are to be handled. Again, this may be particularly important in the case of children in mainstream programs, who may be subject to stringent rules regarding discipline, including suspension. In appropriate circumstances the IEP may override normal school disciplinary practices.

The IEP should discuss issues such as the use of hearing aids and/or auditory trainers (particularly for younger children), seating in the classroom (particularly in mainstream situations), lighting (particularly for children who speechread but also, where appropriate, for children who sign), teacher placement (to ensure, for example, that the teacher does not stand with his or her back to a window, making speechreading impossible), acoustics, the use of interpreters, the use of special resource teachers, and so forth.

Again, these issues should be addressed in *detail.* One court, for example, ruled in 1994 that a school district was required under the IDEA to provide a deaf high school student with a sign language interpreter to assist her during basketball practice [West Virginia ex rel. Lambert v. The West Virginia State Board of Education, 21 IDELR 647 (W. Va. 1994)]. The school had provided interpreters for the student's classes, but claimed it was not required to do so for extracurricular activities. The court disagreed. Had the IEP specified the use of interpreters during extracurricular activities a court dispute could have been avoided.

All special education and related services to be provided to the child should be addressed in specific detail in the IEP. If a child is to have remedial assistance in reading or general tutorial assistance, for example, such assistance should be outlined in detail. If the child's needs require that amplification be provided at school expense (discussed in the next chapter), the school's obligation to provide the means of amplification should be stated in the IEP. The need for all tapes or movies shown to be closed (or open) captioned should also be specified.

Parents may also wish to ensure that the IEP provides mechanisms for coordinating the services provided to the child, and for the child's various teachers, therapists, and counselors to share information among themselves and with the child's parents. By way of example, when a deaf or hard-of-hearing child is in the early grades (kindergarten through fifth grade) and where appropriate when the child is in later grades, the IEP could provide that the child will carry a daily journal, in which teachers, therapists, counselors, and parents will write each day. Each person who works with the child will be required to jot a simple note explaining what the child is working on, what progress was made, what special problems arose, and any other issue worthy of note. That way, everyone will be aware of what other members of the team are doing, and persons involved with the child can coordinate their efforts and work jointly to help the child. Further, the child's parents will be aware of what is going on in school on a daily basis, and can provide appropriate assistance or guidance at home. Parents should note in the journal any special concerns or progress observed at home, which will assist school personnel in providing optimal services to the child.

The IEP should also incorporate the need for the child to develop independence as a person who is deaf or hard-of-hearing. Thus, for example, the IEP for children in early grades might specify what year the child is to learn how to put on, take off and/or adjust his or her hearing aid and/or FM system, or to let his or her teacher know when new batteries for hearing devices are required. In later grades, the IEP may address the child's need to know how to seek assistance from teachers when extra help is required or how and when to ask questions in class without inviting embarrassment. An IEP for a high school student might address the student's need to learn how to explain his or her hearing loss to classmates, to reach out and make friends despite communication barriers, and/or to understand the purpose of IEP meetings and how to actively participate in such meetings.

It is of crucial importance that the IEP be sufficiently detailed to ensure that both the school district and the parents are clearly aware of the child's needs, the explicit services that will be provided to the child, and the expected results of the services provided.

Question: **Once the parents and educators have agreed on the substance of the IEP to be developed for the child, and once the IEP document is drafted, do the responsibilities of parents end with respect to development of their child's educational program for that year?**

Answer: No. Parental involvement must continue throughout the school year. Ultimately, it is the parents' responsibility to ensure that their deaf or hard-of-hearing child is obtaining an appropriate education. Parents of young children should visit their child's classroom at regular intervals throughout the year. Parents of children of all ages should review their child's homework (if any) and written work performed during school on a daily basis, and should review their child's progress (via discussions with both the child and the child's teachers) on a regular basis.

It is up to parents to monitor the educational setting to ensure that their child's IEP is being properly carried out, both procedurally and substantively. At the first indication of a problem parents should intervene, in a pleasant and cooperative manner, to ensure that the difficulty is resolved immediately, before a minor problem escalates into a major problem. (Where older children are involved, parental involvement may simply take the form of providing guidance to assist the child in resolving the problem himself or herself.)

Parents are often worried about being viewed as "troublemakers" or as wrongfully interfering in the educational setting. If parents approach school personnel in a pleasant manner, and are as cooperative as possible without forfeiting their goals, this should not be a concern. In some cases parents of deaf and hard-of-hearing children should worry less about what educators think of them and more about assuming an active role in their child's educational program. Often it is the parents who make the difference between a quality educational experience for their child and an educational experience that does not provide the child with appropriate benefits.

Question: **What happens to the child if the parents and school district cannot agree on the appropriate placement for the child, or when the school district plans to change the child's educational placement or program and the parents do not agree? Where will the child be placed pending resolution of the dispute?**

Answer: Under the "stay put" rule, the child is to remain in his or her "present educational current placement" pending resolution of a *placement* dispute. This means that the child must remain in the placement in which the child was being educated prior to the onset of the current placement dispute. If the dispute has to do with the child's initial placement in school, if the parents consent the child will be placed in the regular public school program until the dispute is resolved. It is important to understand, however, that parents always have the right to remove their child from the public school and place the child in private school or some other educational setting. Thus, the stay put provision operates to prevent the *school district* from unilaterally (by themselves, without the parents' consent) changing the child's placement.

Notwithstanding the stay put provision, the school district and the parents may always agree to change the child's placement pending resolution of the dispute.

The stay put provision applies only when *placement* disputes are at issue. It does not apply when parents and school district are in dispute about changes in the child's *program* rather than the child's placement. Changes in program include such factors as transfer to a different building, a change in transportation arrangements, changes in the location of the school, and so forth.

The Department of Education takes the position that, when a school district closes a school, there is no change of placement if a child with a disability is provided with the same educational services and opportunities for interaction with nondisabled children at another location. In one case, however, the court held that providing a deaf child with special education services in a program at a local public school, rather than the residential school for the deaf that the child formerly attended, constituted a change in placement triggering the stay put provision [Brimmer v. Traverse City Area Public Schools, 872 F. Supp. 447, 22 IDELR 5 (W.D. Mich. 1994)].

The placement versus program issue revolves around the question of whether the proposed change will substantially or significantly affect the services and programs being provided to the child. If so, a change of placement is proposed rather than a change of program. Unfortunately, courts have viewed the removal of a deaf child from an oral setting and placement in a total communication setting, or vice versa, as a change in program and not a change in placement.

When the dispute involves a change in placement, the stay put provision provides that before making such change the school district must follow IDEA procedural requirements (such as providing notice to the parents and an opportunity for the parents to participate in the formulation of a new IEP for their child).

CHAPTER 3

Appropriate Education

This chapter addresses the "appropriate" education to which every deaf and hard-of-hearing child is entitled under the IDEA. The legal standard for an "appropriate education" is explained, and the question of what services and/or auxiliary aids must be provided to assist a deaf or hard-of-hearing child in obtaining an appropriate education is discussed at length. The necessity (or lack thereof) of placement options, in terms of both location and methods of teaching, is addressed. Recommendations are provided to assist parents in ensuring that their deaf and hard-of-hearing children are taught in the parents' chosen communication mode(s).

Question: **What does it mean to say that a child who is deaf or hard-of-hearing is entitled to an "appropriate" education?**

Answer: The United States Supreme Court has said that an appropriate education for a child with a disability is one that is reasonably calculated to provide the child with sufficient educational benefit [Board of Education of the Hendrick Hudson Central School District v. Rowley, 458 U.S. 176 (1982)]. Under the IDEA the child is NOT entitled to the "*best*" education available, or to the "*most*" appropriate education available. Rather, the child is only entitled to an education that provides sufficient benefit. What constitutes sufficient benefit is to be decided on a case-by-case basis. Obviously that determination is very subjective, and will differ in every case, depending on both the individual circumstances involved and the persons making the decision.

The individual states are free, however, to provide *greater* benefits to students with disabilities than those provided under the IDEA (although the states may not provide fewer or less benefits to such students). A few states, therefore, have enacted laws that provide that students with disabilities are entitled to more than the "meaningful educational benefit" to which they are entitled under the IDEA. Those states require that students with disabilities must be educated in a manner that will allow them to achieve "maximum benefit" from the educational system or to reach their "maximum potential." Courts have held, for example, that Massachusetts, Tennessee, California, and Michigan impose higher standards than the meaningful benefit standard applied under the IDEA.

When a state law imposes a higher standard, that higher standard must be applied, which in some cases will assist parents of children with disabilities. Even when the state has a higher standard of "appropriate" education, however, the least restrictive environment mandate still applies.

Question: **For an educational program to be appropriate for a deaf or hard-of-hearing child, must the school district provide interpreters to ensure that the child hears all that is said in the classroom?**

Answer: In the most significant case decided under the IDEA, Board of Education of the Hendrick Hudson Central School District v. Rowley [458 U.S. 176 (1982)], the United States Supreme Court ruled that Amy Rowley, a deaf student with minimal residual hearing, was not entitled to be provided with an interpreter in the classroom.

Amy Rowley was an excellent speechreader. She was in a regular first grade classroom and had been provided with an FM amplifier. She received instruction from a tutor for deaf children for 1 hour each day and speech therapy for 3 hours per week. Amy was doing very well in school, and was in the upper half of her class, despite the fact that she was only able to understand approximately 50% of what was said in the classroom. Her parents requested that she be provided with a sign language interpreter for her academic classes so that she could hear all that was said. The school refused to provide the interpreter, and ultimately the Supreme Court agreed with the school. The Court held that Amy was receiving sufficient educational benefit from her school program, as evidenced by the fact that she was doing well in school, and thus the school did not have to provide additional assistance.

Since the Rowley case was decided by the Supreme Court, the Court's ruling in that case governs throughout the country. However, it is important to understand that the Supreme Court did not say in Rowley that an interpreter would *never* be required for a deaf child. All the Court said was that an interpreter was not necessary for *Amy* to receive sufficient educational benefit from her school program. In other cases lower courts have held that deaf children could not receive sufficient educational benefit from their educational programs without the assistance of interpreters. In those cases schools were required to provide interpreters. Moreover, in many situations schools have voluntarily provided both sign language and oral interpreters for deaf children, when such services have been deemed necessary to allow the children to obtain meaningful benefit from their educational programs.

Parents who want their child's school district to provide the child with an interpreter, either sign language or oral, must frame their request properly. Parents should simply assert that their child is not able to follow what is being said in the classroom without an interpreter, that the child is not able to keep up with his or her studies without an interpreter, and that the child is suffering (or will suffer, if the child is not yet in school) severe frustration in the classroom without an interpreter. (If the child is already in school and having difficulties, of course, that fact should be asserted in support of the need for an interpreter.)

If a sign language interpreter is requested, parents should explain that the child is more comfortable with signs than speechreading and that the child is more proficient in reading signs than speech. If an oral interpreter is requested, parents should explain that the child does not sign, and that the child is a good speechreader and able to utilize an oral interpreter. In either case it must be emphasized that the interpreter is *necessary* to allow the child to receive meaningful benefit from the classroom—otherwise the child will simply be sitting in class without understanding what is going on.

The request should *not* be framed in terms of the child's need for an interpreter to receive maximum benefit from the classroom setting, because under the IDEA the child is not entitled to receive maximum benefit. (In those few states that do entitle children with disabilities to receive maximum benefit such an argument would be permitted, however.) Further, a request for a sign language interpreter in a regular education classroom should *not* be framed in terms of the child's need to be taught via a different "methodology" (that is, by describing sign language as one "method" of teaching children with hearing losses and auditory/oral communication as another "method"). That was one of the problems that existed in the Rowley case. In Rowley the Supreme Court held that school districts have considerable leeway in deciding issues of "methodology"; thus it is unwise for parents to make that an issue, particularly where it is unnecessary.

Once the need for an interpreter in the classroom is established, it will be easier to show the need for an interpreter at
other school functions, such as during extracurricular activities. Some schools voluntarily provide interpreting assistance
in settings other than the classroom; some courts have ordered schools to provide such interpreting assistance.

Question: **If a child requires a hearing aid or an FM system, and does not have one or both, must the school district provide either or both?**

Answer: If it is determined that, to receive an appropriate
education, a child classified as educationally disabled requires
either or both a hearing aid or an FM system in the classroom,
the school district must provide the necessary equipment
under the IDEA.

Question: **Can the school district require the child's parents to pay for the hearing aid or FM system?**

Answer: No. The IDEA requires that the appropriate education to be provided to a child with a disability must be "free."
If a hearing aid and/or FM is required for the child to receive
an appropriate education, such equipment must be provided
free of charge.

Question: **Does this mean that school districts must pay
for hearing aids for children to wear all the time, at home
as well as in school?**

Answer: No. In most situations a child who is deaf or hard-
of-hearing will have his or her own hearing aid, that he or she
wears all the time. When the child comes to school with that
hearing aid, the child may use that aid in school, or the child
may just use a school-provided auditory trainer. If a child does

not have a hearing aid, however, and requires one to receive an appropriate education, the school district may have to provide one. This decision will be made on a case-by-case basis, looking to all relevant factors relating to the child's situation.

This raises the question of whether the child must be allowed to take a school-purchased hearing aid home at the end of the day. Parents who cannot afford to purchase a hearing aid for use at home may argue that use of the hearing aid on a 24-hour basis is required to provide the child with an appropriate education (since to receive optimum benefit from a hearing aid the child must wear it all the time and become proficient at using his or her residual hearing). The author is not aware of any court or administrative decision addressing this question. Conceivably, however, parents *may* be able to succeed on such a claim.

Question: **How does the Least Restrictive Environment (LRE) mandate relate to the requirement that the child receive an appropriate education?**

Answer: The first priority is to ensure that a child receives an appropriate education. The least restrictive environment (LRE) concept, while important, is secondary. The IDEA requires that a child with a disability be placed in the LRE to the "maximum extent *appropriate.*" Thus, not all children who are deaf or hard-of-hearing are to be educated in a regular education setting, since a regular education setting may not be appropriate for some children with hearing losses. Moreover, the LRE for some deaf and hard-of-hearing children may not be the LRE for other deaf and hard-of-hearing children.

The appropriateness and LRE requirements are heavily intertwined, however, and must be looked at together when determining the placement for a child with a hearing loss. The least restrictive alternative among those placements that have been determined to be appropriate for the child must be chosen.

Question: **What placement options must be available for children who are deaf or hard-of-hearing?**

Answer: Under the IDEA, every school district must ensure that a "continuum of alternative placements" is available to meet the needs of children who are deaf and hard-of-hearing, with respect to special education and related services. This requires that a variety of placements be available, such as placement in a regular classroom with appropriate assistance, placement in a regular classroom for part of the day and special classes for other parts of the day, placement in an oral program for children with hearing losses, placement in a sign language program for children with hearing losses, and residential placement in either an oral or sign language program. A school district must notify parents of its obligation to provide a full continuum of placement options when sending notice of an IEP meeting.

A school district may not refuse to place a child in the least restrictive appropriate placement by simply stating that no such placement exists in the district. The district is obligated to fill a gap in the continuum of alternative placements (if the school district does not fulfill that obligation, the state department of education must do so). Further, placement decisions may NOT be premised on the severity of the child's hearing loss, the availability of "space" for the child in a particular program, the availability of related services in a particular program, or the convenience of the school district.

This does not mean, however, that school districts must offer instruction in every variation of every possible form of oral communication or sign language for students who are deaf or hard-of-hearing. Thus, for example, a court has held that a school district was not required to educate a deaf child via use of a strict SEE (signing exact English) system, but could permissibly utilize a modified SEE system [Petersen v. Hastings Public Schools, 831 F. Supp. 732 (D. Neb. 1993), 20 IDELR 252].

Courts have also held that a school district may coordinate specific programs for children with a particular disability at a central location, rather than offering every type of program at every school. Thus, for example, a court has held that a school district that offered a cued speech program in a centrally located school did not have to duplicate that cued speech program at a child's local school [Barnett v. Fairfax County School Board, 927 F.2d 146 (4th Cir. 1991), 17 EHLR 350]. Similarly, a school district could offer a sign language program at one central school and an oral program at another central school. Sign language and oral programs would not be required to be offered at *every* school.

It is not appropriate, however, for a school district to provide *only* an oral program or *only* a sign language program for all children who are deaf or hard-of-hearing. That would violate the continuum of educational options requirement.

Similarly, if it is found that a child requires cued speech to receive an appropriate education, a school district could not refuse to educate the child via cued speech for the reason that it does not have a cued speech program. To satisfy the continuum of educational options requirement, at a minimum the school district would have to provide the child with a cued speech interpreter. (This assumes, of course, that the parents have succeeded in showing that the child requires cued speech to receive an appropriate education. A school district may argue, for example, that cued speech is not required, but rather that total communication would enable the child to receive an appropriate education.)

Question: **How can parents show that education in a particular communication mode is appropriate for their child? For example, how would parents succeed on their claim that their child requires a sign language program, or an oral program, or a cued-speech program to receive an appropriate education?**

Answer: This is the most difficult question facing parents of children who are deaf or hard-of-hearing. There is no ready answer to this question. Following are some guidelines for parents to follow, however:

First, it must be remembered that the child is only entitled to AN appropriate education, not to the *MOST* appropriate education. Thus, it is important that parents focus on the fact that the program they seek for their child is the appropriate program for their child, while any conflicting program recommended by the school district is not appropriate. Parents should not claim that their preferred program is better than the school district's recommended program, but should claim that the school district's recommended program is not appropriate *at all.*

Second, the courts have refused to become embroiled in controversies involving educational *methodology.* Courts take the position that school administrators, as educational "experts," are in the best position to determine issues of educational methodology. Thus, it is important that parents take pains not to structure the issue of sign language versus auditory/oral communication versus cued speech as one of methodology, but as one involving educational goals and outcomes. Unfortunately, however, courts continue to consider this issue as one of methodology, and it is questionable whether a court could be persuaded to view the issue in any other fashion.

When seeking an oral (or auditory-verbal) program for their child parents should focus on the following goals: (a) ensuring that the child develops appropriate skills (verbal or oral communication, social, and others) necessary to allow full integration into mainstream (hearing) society; and (b) ensuring that maximum postsecondary and educational employment opportunities are available to the child when he or she leaves school (which requires the ability to communicate orally). If the child comes from a hearing family, emphasis should also be placed on the need for the child to communicate orally to be a full-fledged member of his or her family and the family's environment. Parents should stress the need for the child to use the same type of communication at home and in school. Parents can also assert that the child has the right to be taught in the native language of the child's family and country.

Because the IDEA requires that school districts take steps to assist children with disabilities in making the transition from school to the next phase of their lives (such as postsecondary education, trade school, work), parents should stress the need for the child to be able to speak and read English, and to communicate with hearing people, in order to effectively make such a transition.

When seeking a cued speech program for their child parents should focus on similar goals, and explain that their child requires cued speech to assist him or her in the oral communication process that will lead to achievement of those goals.

When seeking a sign language program for their child parents should focus on the following goals: (a) ensuring that the child accepts himself or herself as a Deaf person and takes part in the Deaf world—which is his or her alleged birthright; (b) ensuring that the child will immediately maximize his or her sign language or manual communication skills, which will result in a less frustrating and more comfortable—and thus more successful—educational setting.

In every case the parents must incorporate an argument relating to least restrictive environment (LRE) into this discussion of the appropriate educational placement for their child. In many cases, it may be decided that *either* a manual or oral (or cued speech) program would be appropriate for a child who is deaf or hard-of-hearing, because it is determined that either program is reasonably calculated to provide the child with meaningful educational benefit. In that case, parents are not likely to succeed in overturning the school district's chosen placement unless the parents can show that the school district's proposed placement is not the least restrictive placement among the alternative appropriate placements. The next chapter explains how the least restrictive environment issue should be addressed.

Question: **Who decides what is the appropriate educational placement and/or program for a particular deaf or hard-of-hearing child?**

Answer: The IEP team (including parents) make that decision. If the team cannot agree (i.e., if parents and school administrators disagree), a due process hearing must be conducted, and the hearing officer will make that determination. If the "losing" party in the due process hearing appeals the hearing officer's decision, ultimately the court will make the decision.

CHAPTER 4

Least Restrictive Environment (LRE)

This chapter addresses the legal concept of "least restrictive environment" (LRE). The term is clearly defined and distinguished from other terms and concepts, such as "mainstreaming" and "inclusion." An explanation is provided with respect to the manner in which the LRE concept applies to children who are deaf and hard-of-hearing. Recommendations are provided to assist parents in presenting information relating to LRE in a manner that will help obtain parents' chosen placements for their children. Legal standards for determining the LRE for a given child are addressed.

Question: **Is least restrictive environment (LRE) the same as "mainstreaming"?**

Answer: Mainstreaming refers to the participation of children with disabilities side-by-side with nondisabled children. It can occur in academic classes or elsewhere, such as in the cafeteria, at recess, or during intramural sports. The term "mainstreaming" is often inappropriately used as meaning the same thing as LRE. Mainstreaming, however, is just one example of the application of the LRE principle. The concept of LRE is much broader than mainstreaming. LRE favors mainstreaming for those children for whom it is appropriate, but recognizes that for some children mainstreaming is not the LRE.

Question: Is least restrictive environment (LRE) the same as "inclusion"?

Answer: Inclusion generally refers to educating children with disabilities completely in educational programs for nondisabled children. Inclusion differs from mainstreaming in that a child with a disability in an inclusion program is not expected to keep up academically with the nondisabled children in the class, nor is the child with a disability expected to meet all of the regular educational requirements in order to move to the next grade level. Rather, the child with a disability is to be provided with an adapted curriculum and to be moved to the next grade level if he or she meets the reasonable goals of his or her IEP.

In some circles, the term "inclusion" is held to mean inclusion, or immersion, in a Deaf cultural environment, where the deaf or hard-of-hearing child is immersed in Deaf culture.

Again, the concept of LRE is much broader than inclusion, however the term inclusion is defined. LRE favors inclusion (either in a regular school program or in a Deaf cultural environment) for those children for whom it is appropriate, but recognizes that for some children inclusion (in one or either form) is not appropriate.

In some cases, of course, full mainstreaming (rather than "inclusion" as defined above) is appropriate for a child who is deaf or hard-of-hearing. Under the mainstreaming concept the child will be expected to meet the same educational requirements as other children in the classroom.

Question: **What does the least restrictive environment (LRE) concept mean when applied to a child who is deaf or hard-of-hearing?**

Answer: The LRE for a deaf or hard-of-hearing child is one that best meets the individual needs of the child, taking into consideration all relevant factors. Among the relevant factors to be considered are the communication mode of both the child and his or her family; the child's language level and communication abilities; the child's social skills and needs; the child's personality, including emotional strengths and needs; the unique family situation; the child's educational abilities; and, ultimately, the family's goals and educational objectives for the child.

Question: **If parents wish to place their deaf or hard-of-hearing child in a residential school using oral communication, what factors should the parents emphasize with respect to least restrictive environment (LRE)?**

Answer: The parents should emphasize that: (a) it is the parents' desire that the child learn to communicate orally so that the child can communicate with family members, family friends, and other hearing persons; (b) the child already has some oral communication skills (if this is so); (c) the child's oral skills are not yet adequate to enable the child to achieve satisfactorily in a regular school program; (d) the child requires intensive oral/aural and/or auditory training to develop adequate oral skills; (e) consistency and continuity of goals, expectations, focus, and training of personnel will be present throughout the child's educational program; (f) the child will receive double benefit from socializing with other deaf children while at the same time receiving training that is intended to lead to the ability to socialize with all members of society; and, ultimately, (g) the family's goal is for the child to be able to interact with members of the larger hearing society by communicating orally with such persons.

When asserting the right to an oral (or auditory-verbal) education, the focus should be on the rationale that the goal of education is to prepare the child for life after school. Since the majority of people in this world can hear and communicate orally, an educational goal should be to maximize the child's ability to communicate with hearing people (without having to rely on an intermediary to interpret). Parents should assert that a person who can communicate orally has greater employment opportunities than someone who cannot communicate with people at the workplace.

When comparing placement in a residential oral school to placement in a sign language environment, the LRE concept focuses on long-range planning. The rationale is that, although it may be less restrictive initially if a child who is deaf or hard-of-hearing utilizes sign language, ultimately placement in a sign language environment will lead to a more restrictive environment. When comparing placement in a residential oral school to placement in a regular classroom, the rationale is that it is not less restrictive to place a deaf or hard-of-hearing child in a regular classroom if the child does not have sufficient oral skills to understand what is being said or to communicate his or her own thoughts.

Question: If parents wish to place their deaf or hard-of-hearing child in a residential school using total communication, what factors should the parents emphasize with respect to least restrictive environment (LRE)?

Answer: The parents should emphasize that: (a) it is the parents' desire that their child communicate via sign language; (b) the child currently communicates via sign language (if that is so); (c) the child will develop language faster if placed in an environment where he or she is immersed in sign language that is visible to the child; (d) the child will be happier and/or more emotionally stable if placed in an environment where everyone signs and communication is easier—and less stressful—for the child; (e) the child will have greater social interaction with other children if all the children in his or her class are deaf and the child is not "different" from his or her classmates; (e) the child will benefit from observing deaf role models (i.e., teachers and staff members who are deaf or hard-of-hearing); and, ultimately, (f) the family's goal is for the child to become a part of Deaf society and culture.

The focus should be on the rationale that education in a regular classroom, even with necessary support services such as an interpreter and/or special education services provided by a teacher of the deaf, is more restrictive, rather than less restrictive, for this child. The child will be more isolated (or less integrated) if placed in a regular school program—where the child will have communication difficulties and social problems—than if placed in a school for deaf children.

Question: **If parents wish to place their child in a regular education program with the assistance of a sign language interpreter, what factors should the parents emphasize with respect to LRE?**

Answer: The parents should emphasize that the child is capable of being educated in his or her local school, and will benefit thereby from being at home with his or her family, integrating with the neighborhood children, and receiving optimal educational instruction. This, therefore, is the LRE placement for this child. To succeed in the regular educational program, however, the child requires a sign language interpreter since: (a) the child is not able to follow the teacher and class discussion via speechreading and/or use of residual hearing and (b) the child is more comfortable utilizing sign language than oral modes of communication. In this regard, therefore, a sign language inter-preter is less restrictive for this child than an oral interpreter.

Question: **If parents wish to place their child in a regular education program, with or without the assistance of an oral interpreter, what factors should the parents emphasize with respect to least restrictive environment (LRE)?**

Answer: The parents should make the above arguments (dis-cussed in chapter 3 regarding appropriate education and earli-er in this chapter) with respect to the goals of oral education, and should further argue that placement in the local school is less restrictive than placement in a special program for deaf children utilizing oral communication (again because the child is close to home and is able to integrate with neighborhood [hearing] children). If the child requires an oral interpreter the parents should focus on the facts that (a) the child cannot understand much of what is said in the classroom via an FM system; (b) the child cannot understand much of what is said in the classroom via speechreading without an interpreter because the teacher moves around while talking, faces the blackboard, and so on, and because it is not possible to see the mouths of the students who speak during class discussion; (c) the child does not use sign language, or is not fluent in sign language, but is a good speechreader and is more comfortable utilizing an oral interpreter. In this regard, therefore, an oral interpreter is necessary to allow the child to function in this LRE.

Question: **If parents wish to place their child in a regular education program with the assistance of a cued speech interpreter, what factors should the parents emphasize with respect to least restrictive environment (LRE)?**

Answer: The same basic rationale used when arguing for an oral interpreter applies.

Question: **What standards do the courts apply when determining what constitutes the least restrictive environment (LRE) for a particular child?**

Answer: As previously explained, the IDEA requires children with disabilities to be educated with children without disabilities to the maximum extent appropriate. In accord with this premise, under the IDEA children with disabilities are to be removed from the regular educational environment only when education in regular classes cannot be satisfactorily achieved even if supplementary aids and services are provided. The courts have applied different standards when interpreting this requirement, including the following:

The Sixth Circuit Court of Appeals (which governs cases arising in Kentucky, Michigan, Ohio, and Tennessee) applied a so-called "portability" test in the 1983 case of <u>Roncker v. Walter</u> [700 F.2d 1058 (6th Cir. 1983), <u>cert. denied</u>, 464 U.S. 864 (1983)]. Under that test, if the particular service that makes a more restrictive setting appropriate can be transported to a less restrictive setting, the services must be provided for the child in the less restrictive setting. If, for example, a special school for deaf children was felt to be the appropriate placement for a deaf or hard-of-hearing child simply because that school was equipped to provide speech therapy to the child while the child's neighborhood school did not offer speech therapy, under this test the speech therapy services would have to be provided at the local school, which is the least restrictive environment for the child. If, however, the reason the special school is deemed appropriate for the child with a hearing loss is because the child requires immersion in a constant speech program (which is part of the special school), and if that setting cannot be transferred to the local school, then the local school would not be the appropriate placement for the child.

The Fifth Circuit United States Court of Appeals (which governs cases arising in Louisiana, Mississippi, and Texas) has refused to follow the Sixth Circuit's portability test. In the 1989 case of Daniel R.R. v. State Board of Education [874 F.2d 1036 (5th Cir. 1989), 15 EHLR 441:433], the Fifth Circuit devised its own two-pronged test. Under the first prong the court must ask whether education in the regular classroom can be satisfactorily achieved if the child is provided with supplemental aids and services. The court must determine whether the school district is providing sufficient supplemental aids and services and is modifying its educational program to an adequate extent to meet the needs of the child. If the school is not fulfilling that obligation, the school must do so before it can remove the child from the regular class-room. If the school is fulfilling that obligation, but the child cannot receive an appropriate education in the regular classroom, it must then be determined whether the school has mainstreamed the child to the maximum extent appropriate.

The Third Circuit United States Court of Appeals (which governs cases arising in Delaware, New Jersey, and Pennsylvania) agreed with the Fifth Circuit's Daniel R.R. test in the 1993 case of Oberti v. Board of Education of the Borough of Clementon School District [995 F.2d 1204 (3rd Cir. 1993), 19 IDELR 908]. Further, the Third Circuit held that since the IDEA places great emphasis on the integration of children with disabilities into the regular educational system, a school district bears the burden of proving that a child with a disability should not be educated in the regular classroom.

The Ninth Circuit Court of Appeals (which governs cases arising in Alaska, Arizona, California, Hawaii, Idaho, Montana, Nevada, Oregon, and Washington) applied an even different test in the 1994 case of Sacramento Unified School District v. Holland [14 F.3d 1398 (9th Cir. 1994), 20 IDELR 812], which is characterized as a hybrid of the Sixth Circuit's Roncker test and the Fifth Circuit's Daniel R. test. Under the Ninth Circuit's test four factors must be considered and balanced when deciding whether a child with a disability should be educated in a regular class-room: (a) the educational benefits of full-time placement in a regular class; (b) the nonacademic benefits of placement in a regular class; (c) the effect the child will have on the teacher and the children in the regular class; and (d) the cost of main-streaming the child with a disability.

As these examples illustrate, the courts apply a variety of standards when determining what constitutes the LRE for a child with a disability. Unfortunately, there is no one "magic" test that parents can rely upon. The result may differ depending upon the state in which the family resides (which determines the test or standard that will apply), as well as subjective factors that are unique to each individual situation.

In 1992, the DOE issued a policy guidance with respect to the LRE issue, suggesting that when developing an IEP for a child who is deaf, numerous factors should be considered, including the child's:

1. Communication needs and the child's and family's preferred mode of communication;
2. Linguistic needs;
3. Severity of hearing loss and potential for using residual hearing;
4. Academic level; and
5. Social, emotional, and cultural needs, including opportunities for peer instructions and communication. [19 IDELR 463]

The policy guidance notes that school districts should not **presume** that children who are deaf should be placed in regular classroom settings, but recognizes that regular educational settings are appropriate to meet the needs of some students who are deaf. Each case must be decided on an individual basis.

Question: **Doesn't the IDEA require that children with disabilities be educated as close to home as possible?**

Answer: The Department of Education's (DOE's) IDEA regulations do provide that a school district should ensure that the educational placement of a child with a disability is as close as possible to the child's home. As with other aspects of the least restrictive environment (LRE) principle, however, the primary concern is to provide an appropriate education for the child. Thus, if the neighborhood school cannot provide the child with an appropriate education, the school district is not necessarily required to place the child in the neighborhood school. Further, as discussed earlier in this book, the concept of placing a child with a disability as close to home as possible does not override the school district's ability to exercise discretion to utilize resources in an efficient manner. School districts may concentrate resources for children with particular needs and/or disabilities at specified schools.

Question: Who decides what is the least restrictive environment (LRE) for a particular deaf or hard-of-hearing child?

Answer: Again, the IEP team makes that decision. If the team cannot reach an agreement (i.e., if the parents and school district disagree), a due process hearing must be held, in which case the hearing officer will make the decision. If the hearing officer's decision is appealed by the "losing" party (the party whose position is rejected by the hearing officer), ultimately the court will make the decision.

Question: In a state in which separate money is set aside for special programs or schools for educating deaf or hard-of-hearing children, can a school district claim that a deaf or hard-of-hearing child must attend one of those special schools or programs for budgetary reasons?

Answer: No. The 1997 Amendments to the IDEA provide that a state cannot use a funding mechanism distributing state funds on the basis of the type of setting in which a child with a disability must be served if that funding mechanism would violate the LRE rule (i.e., that a child with a disability must be educated with nondisabled children unless the severity of the child's disability prevents such education).

CHAPTER 5

Related Services

This chapter discusses additional services, other than the traditional educational services provided in a classroom setting, that must be provided to assist a deaf or hard-of-hearing child to obtain an appropriate education. Both the type of services to be provided and issues relating to the cost of and payment for such services are addressed.

Question: **What related services must be provided for children who are deaf or hard-of-hearing?**

Answer: School districts must provide whatever services are necessary to enable a deaf or hard-of-hearing child to receive an appropriate education. In different circumstances necessary related services might include speech therapy, auditory training, provision of an interpreter or an interpreter/aide, provision of a resource teacher, provision of tutorial assistance, provision of notetakers, provision of sign language training for the child or for the child and his or her parents, transportation services, rehabilitation counseling services, captioned video tapes, TTYs for telephone use, and so forth. Because assistive technology services must be made available when necessary to provide an appropriate education, special equipment, such as an FM system or other assistive listening device, will need to be provided where appropriate. As previously discussed, if assistive technology (such as a hearing aid) is required for home use to provide a child with a free appropriate public education, the school district may have to provide such technology for home use. The Office of Special Education Services takes the position that the purchase of personal hearing aids must be decided on a case-to-case basis, which is in accord with the IDEA's focus on individual needs.

The definition of the term "related services" in the IDEA is open-ended. Thus, while the IDEA lists examples of specific related services, those examples are not the only related services that school districts may be required to provide. Whatever services are necessary to ensure that the child receives an appropriate education must be provided.

Question: If a deaf or hard-of-hearing child attends a school outside the boundary of his or her neighborhood school district, and that school is held to be the appropriate placement for the child, must the child's neighborhood school district pay to transport the child to and from that school?

Answer: Yes. Because the IDEA lists transportation as a specified form of related service, courts have held that a school district must transport a child with a disability to and from school even when the school the child attends is outside the geographical boundaries of the school district.

Question: Must a school district ever provide the child's parents with transportation services?

Answer: In some circumstances, yes. If the child's IEP provides that services (such as sign language training) must be provided to the parents to enable the child to receive an appropriate education, transporting the parents to such services (such as sign language classes) could be considered a necessary related service. In such a situation, however, the need for transportation would probably have to be shown to be specifically related to the unique needs caused by the child's hearing loss (this test would clearly be satisfied where sign language training for parents was at issue, for example).

Question: **If, to receive an appropriate education, a child requires a hearing aid or assistive listening device, to be used either at school only or both at school and at home, must the school district assume full responsibility for fitting and caring for the device?**

Answer: Yes. The IDEA requires school districts to provide assistive technology services as well as assistive technology devices. The term "assistive technology services" is defined as including "selecting, designing, fitting, customizing, adapting, applying, maintaining, repairing, or replacing of assistive technology devices" [20 U.S.C. § 1401(a)(26)(C)].

Question: **If the child and/or his or her family must receive training to learn how to use an assistive listening device or other assistive technology device, must the school district provide such training?**

Answer: Yes. The IDEA provides that assistive listening services which must be provided where necessary include training or technical assistance for the student and, where necessary, the student's family. The IDEA further provides that such training or technical assistance must be provided to educators and other school personnel, including persons providing rehabilitation services, where necessary.

Question: **May parents be required to utilize their health insurance benefits to pay for necessary related services for their child?**

Answer: Parents may voluntarily utilize their insurance benefits, or permit school districts to access their insurance benefits, to pay for related services. If parents voluntarily choose to access their private insurance benefits for such purposes, an insurance company cannot refuse to accept financial responsibility by claiming that the IDEA requires the school district to pay for such services. (If the insurance proceeds only pay for part of the services, the school district would be required to pay the remaining portion of the cost.)

Parents may not be *required* to make their insurance benefits available for services for their deaf or hard-of-hearing children, however, if the parents would incur any financial loss in doing so. Financial losses include, but are not limited to: (a) a decrease in available coverage or benefit under the insurance policy (for example, if insurance benefits are utilized to pay for counseling and as a result the amount of insurance benefits available for counseling is reduced); (b) an increase in premiums or discontinuation of the policy as a result of the expenditure; and (c) an out-of-pocket expense to the parents, such as payment of a deductible amount incurred when the parents file a claim.

School districts cannot make the provision of special education services conditional on the filing of an insurance claim (including a Medicaid claim). Further, if parents refuse to file an insurance claim, even where doing so would not result in any financial loss to the parents, the school district remains obligated to provide the child with a FAPE.

Question: **May school districts seek reimbursement from Medicaid for expenditures related to the provision of related services?**

Answer: Some state Medicaid plans provide for coverage for services of the type provided as related services under the IDEA. To the extent that Medicaid payment is available under a state plan for such services, Medicaid will be available to reimburse educational agencies for the cost of related services. This situation is outside the scope of parental concern, however.

CHAPTER 6

Private Schooling

This chapter addresses issues relating to children who are deaf or hard-of-hearing and who attend private schools (both religious and nonreligious). Topics addressed include (a) the right of parents to send their children to private schools, (b) situations in which public school districts will or will not be required to pay private school tuition for deaf or hard-of-hearing students, and (c) situations in which public school districts will or will not be required to pay for related services to be provided for deaf or hard-of-hearing children attending private schools. Also addressed are the obligations of private schools toward students who are deaf and hard-of-hearing.

Question: **If a school district cannot appropriately place a child who is deaf or hard-of-hearing in a public program, will the district be required to pay the cost of tuition and related services for that child at a private school?**

Answer: Yes. School districts are responsible for providing a free appropriate public education to each child with a disability. If the district is unable to provide the requisite FAPE in a public school setting (either in the child's local school or another public school), it must pay for appropriate educational services (including related services) to be provided privately. This applies to both

59

nonresidential and residential private schools. Thus, if private residential placement is required to provide the child with an appropriate education, the school district must pay for such placement.

Question: If parents are not satisfied with the educational program designed by their local school district, may they choose to place their deaf or hard-of-hearing child in a private school (even one that does not meet state requirements with respect to the education of children with disabilities)?

Answer: Yes. Although every school district/local education agency must be prepared to provide a FAPE to every child with a disability residing in its jurisdiction, parents of such children are not required to accept an offered placement. Parents may choose instead to place their child in a private school, even if the school does not meet state standards for the education of children with disabilities.

If parents plan to seek reimbursement from the school district for the cost of such private schooling, however, they must follow required procedures, as explained in the responses to the next questions.

Question: If parents do place their deaf or hard-of-hearing child in private school must the school district/local education agency pay for the tuition at the private school?

Answer: If the school district can provide an appropriate education for the child, it will not be required to pay the cost of tuition for the child to attend a private school. The 1997 Amendments to the IDEA, as well as the Department of Education's (DOE's) IDEA regulations, provide that the local school district is not required to pay for the education of a child with a disability at a private school when the school district offers an appropriate placement.

An educational program designed by a school district may be held to be "legally" appropriate for a deaf or hard-of-hearing child even though the child's parents do not agree with the program. As explained later in this text (see chapter 8), however, parents may challenge a school district's determination that it can provide an appropriate education for their child.

If the parents ultimately succeed on their claim, and the school district's proposed program is held *not* to be appropriate, the parents will be entitled to reimbursement of tuition at the private school, assuming that the private school is found to be an appropriate placement for the child. The United States Supreme Court has held that, if the private placement selected by the parents is found to be appropriate and the school district's proposed placement to be inappropriate, the school district must pay for the private placement even if the private school does not meet state standards or is not on a list of "state approved" schools [Florence County School District Four v. Carter, 114 S. Ct. 361 (1993)].

Question: What must parents do to obtain reimbursement from their child's school district for private school expenses?

Answer: The 1997 Amendments to the IDEA provide that in order to obtain reimbursement for private school expenses, parents must have complied with the following requirements:

1. At the last IEP meeting prior to removing their child from public school, the parents must inform the IEP team that they are rejecting the school district's proposed placement and intend to place their child in private school.

ALTERNATIVELY:

Ten business days (including holidays occurring on business days) before removing their child from public school the parents must provide the school with *written* notice of their decision to place the child in private school.

Parents MUST follow one of the above two options or they will be denied reimbursement for private school expenses.

2. If the school district provides the parents with notice of the district's intent to evaluate the child, the parents must make the child available for such evaluation or the parents may not recover reimbursement for private school expenses.

In addition, if a court finds that the parents acted unreasonably in unilaterally placing their child in private school, reimbursement for private school expenses will be denied.

Question: **Even if a child's school district does not pay for tuition at a private school, must the school district pay for related services necessary to allow the child to receive an appropriate education at the private school?**

Answer: The Department of Education's (DOE's) regulations, effective until this book went to press, provide generally that school districts shall make necessary services available to children with disabilities who attend private schools. The DOE has interpreted its regulation narrowly, to permit school districts to refuse to provide related services to children with disabilities attending private schools. According to the DOE, when deciding whether to provide a private school student with a disability with related services, a school district may consider the amount of money available and the relative needs of both public and private school children residing in the district's jurisdiction. According to the DOE, therefore, a school district may refuse to provide services such as interpreters, speech or auditory therapy, or even assistive listening devices, to children with hearing losses whose parents unilaterally place them in private schools.

Some courts have disagreed with the DOE's position. In the 1992 case of Tribble v. Montgomery County Board of Education [798 F. Supp. 668 (M.D. Ala. 1992), 19 IDELR 102], a federal district court in the Middle District of Alabama ruled that under the IDEA a child with a disability is entitled to receive related services from the LEA regardless of whether the student enters the school district's proposed program or is placed in a private school selected by the parents. The court held that the IDEA and its implementing regulations clearly require children with disabilities to receive necessary related services at public expense. Unfortunately, the district court's decision in Tribble was vacated by the Eleventh Circuit United States Court of Appeals after the parties to that action settled their dispute (thus the case was over).

More recently, several federal courts have followed reasoning similar to that in Tribble. The leading case taking that position was K.R. v. Anderson Community School Corporation, 887 F. Supp. 1217 (S.D. Ind. 1995) (subsequently reversed as discussed later in this response). K.R. v. Anderson involved a child with multiple disabilities who needed a full-time instructional assistant to benefit from an educational program, regardless of whether she attended public or private school. The district court held that under the IDEA regulations the school district was required to provide the instructional assistant at the private school at which the child was unilaterally enrolled by her parents. The district court held that under the IDEA "a disabled child and her parents should have essentially the same practical choice between the local public school and a private parochial school that a child without special needs would have" (887 F. Supp. at 1217).

Several courts followed the reasoning of the district court in K.R. v. Anderson, including: Cefalu v. East Baton Rouge Parish School Board and the State of Louisiana, 22 IDELR 1045 (M.D. La. 1995) (the court ordered the school district to provide a full time sign language interpreter for a deaf child unilaterally enrolled by her parents in a private school); Russman v. Board of Education of the Enlarged City School District of the City of Watervliet, 22 IDELR ¶ 1028 (N.D. N.Y. 1995), aff'd, 24 IDELR ¶ 274 (2d Cir. 1996) (the court ordered the school district to provide a child with mental retardation with a part-time consultant teacher, a teaching aide, and speech and occupational therapy at the private school at which she was unilaterally enrolled by her parents; Fowler v. Unified School District No. 259, 23 IDELR ¶ 323 (D. Kan. 1995) (the court ordered the school district to provide a deaf child unilaterally enrolled in private school with one-on-one interpreter services).

Subsequently, however, the decision in K.R. v. Anderson was reversed on appeal [23 IDELR ¶ 1137 (7th Cir. 1996)]. The Seventh Circuit agreed with the position taken by the DOE, and held that under the IDEA school districts may consider their own financial resources in deciding whether to provide services to a child with a disability who is unilaterally enrolled in private school by her parents, and may take into account the number and location of children with disabilities enrolled in private schools. The Seventh Circuit held that when school districts do provide benefits to children with disabilities unilaterally enrolled in private schools, the benefits provided must be comparable to the benefits provided for public school students. Whether to provide those services at the private school in the first instance, however, is left to the school district's discretion. According to the Seventh Circuit, the IDEA regulations do not require that children with disabilities attending private school voluntarily be provided with full benefits. Thus, the Seventh Circuit held that the school did not have to provide the multiply disabled student with a full-time instructional aide at her private school.

Following the Seventh Circuit's decision in K.R. v. Anderson, the Second Circuit affirmed the district court's decision in the

Russman case (discussed above). (The Second Circuit's opinion is found at Russman v. Sobol, 24 IDELR ¶ 274 (2d Cir. 1996).) The Second Circuit disagreed with the Seventh Circuit's reasoning in K.R. v. Anderson, and upheld the district court's ruling in Russman ordering the school district to provide the student with mental retardation with a teaching consultant and teaching aide at the private school.

Two other U.S. courts of appeals have ruled on this issue. The Tenth Circuit decided the appeal of Fowler v. Unified School District No. 259, 25 IDELR ¶ 454 (10th Cir. 1997). Like the Second Circuit, the Tenth Circuit also did *not* follow the Seventh Circuit's reasoning in K.R. v. Anderson. Rather, the Tenth Circuit ruled that the IDEA requires a school district to pay for an interpreter for a deaf child in private schools—up to, and not exceeding, the average cost the district would incur to provide interpreting services to a deaf student in the public schools.

In addition, the Fifth Circuit decided the appeal of Cefalu v. East Baton Rouge Parish School Board, 105 F.3d 393 (5th Cir. 1997). The Fifth Circuit held that: (a) the IDEA is intended to ensure that students voluntarily enrolled in private schools have "a genuine opportunity for equitable participation" in services and programs provided under that Act; and (b) private school students are eligible to receive similar services under the IDEA as those received by similarly situated students in public schools. However, the Fifth Circuit ruled that the disabled student in private school must show genuine need for services at the private school, based on more than mere convenience. If such a showing is made, the public school district must provide services at the private school *unless* the district can show either an economic or noneconomic justifiable reason for denying such services. If the school district makes some showing of a justifiable reason, the student must then show that the school district's position contravenes the IDEA, is not rational, or is otherwise arbitrary.

The Fifth Circuit ruled that in <u>Cefalu</u> the record did not show why the school district had refused to provide an interpreter for the deaf student enrolled in private school. Absent such evidence, the Fifth Circuit held that it could not determine whether the school district complied with the IDEA in denying the student interpreter services. The Circuit Court of appeals sent the case back to the district court to obtain the necessary evidence and act upon that evidence.

Clearly, the courts are in controversy. To resolve this controversy somewhat, the 1997 Amendments to the IDEA attempt to reach a compromise. The 1997 Amendments provide that the amount of money a school district must allocate for special education and related services to be provided to or for children with disabilities unilaterally enrolled in private schools shall equal a "proportionate amount" of federal funds available to that school district for the education of children with disabilities. Thus, for example, suppose 300 children with disabilities (covered under the IDEA) reside in "X" school district. Suppose also that 30 of those 300 children with disabilities, or 10%, are unilaterally placed by their parents in private schools. Ten percent of the federal money allocated to X school district for the education of those 300 children must be allocated for necessary services for the 30 children unilaterally enrolled in private schools. (Note that the 1997 Amendments do not obligate school districts to spend state monies to provide children unilaterally enrolled in private schools with special education and related services.)

Question: **If a deaf or hard-of-hearing child is attending a private school that is operated by a religious entity (a sectarian school), would it violate the United States Constitution for the local school district to provide services to the child on the premises of the sectarian school?**

Answer: The concern with respect to services provided to students in sectarian schools involves the constitutional prohibition against the establishment of religion set forth in the First Amendment. This prohibition, called the "establishment clause," is intended to ensure the separation of church and state.

In Zobrest v. Catalina Foothills School District [113 S. Ct. 52 (1993)] the United States Supreme Court held in 1993 that it did not violate the First Amendment for a public school district to pay for the services of a sign language interpreter for a deaf student attending a parochial school. The Court recognized that a sign language interpreter does not perform the same type of functions as a teacher or a guidance counselor. Although it would violate the establishment clause if the state paid the teacher or guidance counselor to teach or counsel the student on the premises of the sectarian school, the same principle does not apply with respect to the interpreter. An interpreter acts simply as a conduit to further communication. (Note, however, that the Supreme Court did not rule on the issue of whether school districts are *required* to pay for *any* related services provided to children unilaterally placed in private schools.)

Whether the ruling of Zobrest will be held to apply with respect to services other than interpreting services is unclear. In other, earlier cases (not involving children with disabilities) the Supreme Court has held that services that are "therapeutic" or "remedial" cannot be provided at state expense on the premises of a religious school, since to do so would involve excessive entanglement between church and state. Under this reasoning state provision of a special education teacher or a tutor for a student with a hearing loss on the premises of a sectarian school would violate the First Amendment. Arguably, however, services such as speech or auditory training should fall under the rationale of Zobrest, and be permissible.

After the Supreme Court's ruling in Zobrest, in 1994 the DOE's Office of Special Education Programs (OSEP) ruled that it would not violate the First Amendment for a public school district to pay for an FM amplification device for a child with a hearing loss who was attending a parochial school. (OSEP reiterated the DOE's position that the IDEA does not *require* the school district to provide the amplification device for the private school student, however.)

The 1997 Amendments to the IDEA provide that school districts may provide special education and related services to children with disabilities on the premises of a private school, including parochial schools, as "consistent with the law."

Question: **Would it violate the United States Constitution for a public school district to pay for a deaf or hard-of-hearing student to be transported to and from a sectarian school?**

Answer: No. In a case decided before <u>Zobrest</u>, and not involving a child with a disability, the Supreme Court held that publicly funded transportation of sectarian school students does not violate the First Amendment.

Question: **If it were held to violate the Constitution for a state to provide a particular service (such as tutoring assistance) for a deaf or hard-of-hearing student attending a parochial school, could the state pay for such services to be provided at another setting?**

Answer: Yes. First Amendment principles do not apply when services are to be provided at a neutral site off the premises of the sectarian school.

Question: **Is there any law that requires private schools to provide special services for children who are deaf or hard-of-hearing?**

Answer: Private schools that are not affiliated with a religious institution are governed by Title III of the Americans with Disabilities Act (ADA). Title III of the ADA is found at volume 42 of the United States Code, sections 12181–12189 [42 U.S.C. §§ 12181-12189]. Schools affiliated with a religious entity are not covered by Title III of the ADA.

Question: **What are the obligations of private schools toward deaf and hard-of hearing children under Title III of the Americans with Disabilities Act (ADA)? Must a private school that has no religious affiliation prepare an Individualized Education Program (IEP) for a child who is deaf or hard-of-hearing to ensure the child an appropriate education?**

Answer: A private school governed by Title III of the ADA (that is, a private school that has no religious affiliation) has no obligation to provide a deaf or hard-of-hearing child with an appropriate education or to implement an IEP for the child. Under Title III, however, private schools are not permitted to discriminate against students or prospective students on the basis of disability. Thus a private school (that is not religiously affiliated) may not refuse to admit an applicant who is deaf or hard-of-hearing because of the applicant's hearing loss, nor may such a school treat a deaf or hard-of hearing student in a discriminatory fashion.

To avoid discrimination, Title III of the ADA requires a covered private school to provide a deaf or hard-of-hearing student with "reasonable accommodations" to allow the student to participate fully in the school's program. An accommodation is not reasonable if it would: (a) pose an undue financial or administrative burden upon the school or (b) fundamentally change the nature of the school's program.

Unfortunately, the terms "reasonable accommodation" and "undue burden" are not clearly defined. Thus, it will have to be decided on a case-by-case basis whether requested accommodations are reasonable. When a deaf child seeks to have a private school provide him or her with a full-time interpreter, for example, it would have to be decided whether the cost of the interpreter would be unduly burdensome to the school. Given the very tight budgets of many private schools, it is likely that in many cases that cost would be held to be unduly burdensome.

CHAPTER 7

Discipline

This chapter addresses the concept of discipline as it applies to children in public schools who are deaf and hard-of-hearing. The discussion includes the extent to which, and circumstances under which, such children may be suspended or expelled from school, as well as disciplinary matters applicable to situations involving the possession of weapons or drugs. Because the issue of discipline is tangential to the major purpose of this book, the topic is covered only briefly.

Question: **Does the IDEA come into play when the discipline of a deaf or hard-of-hearing child is at issue?**

Answer: Yes. The so-called "stay put" provision in the IDEA prohibits a school district from unilaterally changing the educational placement of a child with a disability. When the placement of a child with a disability is to be changed, IDEA procedural requirements (such as notice to the parents and an opportunity to participate in the formulation of a new IEP for their child) must be followed. In the event of a dispute between parents and the school district regarding the change in placement, the school district must allow the child to "stay put" in his or her current educational placement until resolution of the dispute (dispute resolution is discussed in chapter 8 of this text).

In the 1988 case of <u>Honig v. Doe</u> [448 U.S. 305 (1988)] the United States Supreme Court held that a school district's unilateral expulsion of students with disabilities constitutes a change in placement that cannot be instituted without compliance with the IDEA procedural requirements. Further, the Court held that a suspension for more than 10 days constitutes a change in placement, thus triggering the stay put provision. Under the Supreme Court's ruling, therefore, a school district may temporarily suspend a student with a disability for up to 10 school days. A school district may not suspend the child for more than 10 days, however, without such a temporary suspension being considered a change in placement pursuant to which parents must participate in the decision as to what, if any, changes are to be made to the child's IEP.

The 1997 Amendments to the IDEA incorporate this principle.

Question: Are there any exceptions to this "10-day" rule?

Answer: Yes. The 1997 Amendments to the IDEA provide that a child with a disability may be transferred to an alternate educational setting for up to 45 days if: (a) The child carries a weapon to school or to a school function; or (b) the child knowingly possesses, uses, or offers to sell an illegal drug at school or a school function. During this period the child will be placed in an interim alternative educational program determined by the IEP team.

Question: What happens after a child who is deaf or hard-of-hearing is suspended or expelled for up to 10 days for misbehavior or for up to 45 days for weapon or drug abuses?

Answer: Within 10 days of taking the disciplinary action, the school district must convene an IEP meeting to develop a plan to address the child's behavior.

Question: If a child has not violated a weapon or drug rule, but the school district feels that the behavior of a child who

is deaf or hard-of-hearing is substantially likely to result in injury to the child or others if the child remains in his or her current educational placement, does the district have any options?

Answer: Yes. To assist school districts when they fear that a child's behavior is dangerous, the 1997 Amendments provide that the school district may apply to a due process hearing officer for assistance. The hearing officer may order the child placed in an interim alternative educational placement for up to 45 days if the hearing officer:

1. Finds that the child is substantially likely to injure him/herself or others; and
2. considers the appropriateness of the child's current placement; and
3. determines that the school district has made reasonable efforts to minimize the risk of harm in the child's current placement; and
4. finds that the interim alternative educational placement will enable the child to participate in the general educational setting and receive the services outlined in the child's IEP, and will include services and modifications designed to prevent recurrence of the misbehavior.

If the behavior can be addressed in the child's current educational placement, the child cannot be moved.

Question: **Absent the "dangerousness" type of situation described above, what must a school district do before it can suspend or expel a child who is deaf or hard-of-hearing from school for more than 10 days?**

Answer: First, the school district must notify the child's parents of the district's intent to seek a longer suspension or expulsion, and provide the parents with notice of their procedural rights under the IDEA, as previously explained in this book.

Second, no later than 10 days after the decision to suspend or expel the child for longer than 10 days is made, the school district must hold an IEP meeting to determine whether the child's misbehavior is a manifestation of his or her hearing disability.

Question: How is it determined whether the child's misbehavior is a manifestation of his or her hearing disability?

Answer: The IEP team must consider all relevant factors, including evaluation and diagnostic results, information received from the child's parents, observations of the child, and the child's IEP and placement.

Question: If it is found that the child's misbehavior is not a manifestation of his or her hearing loss what may the school do?

Answer: The school district may follow the same disciplinary procedures it would follow if the child were not disabled, including suspending or expelling the child for more than 10 days.

Question: If it is found that the child's misbehavior IS a manifestation of his or her hearing loss what may the school do?

Answer: The school district may not subject the child to disciplinary action.

Question: In either case, must the school district continue to provide the child with educational services?

Answer: Yes. The 1997 Amendments to the IDEA provide that a child with a disability must be provided with alternative educational services when suspended or expelled, even if that suspension or expulsion is not related to the child's disability.

Question: **If a school district determines that a child's misbehavior is not a manifestation of his or her hearing loss, and thus decides to expel the child or suspend the child from his or her current educational placement for more than 10 days, what can parents do if they disagree with that decision?**

Answer: Parents can request a due process hearing (which is explained in chapter 8 of this book). The 1997 Amendments to the IDEA provide that in this situation the hearing shall be expedited, and thus held promptly.

Question: **What will happen to the child pending resolution of the hearing at which the parents protest a finding that the child's misbehavior was not a manifestation of his or her disability?**

Answer: The 1997 Amendments to the IDEA provide that the child will stay in the interim alternative educational setting for a maximum of 45 days unless the parents and school district agree otherwise.

CHAPTER 8

Dispute Resolution

This chapter addresses actions that may be taken when parents and school district officials are not in agreement with respect to an aspect of the education to be provided for a deaf or hard-of-hearing child. Mediation and administrative and judicial resolution of disputes are addressed. Procedures and policies to be followed are described in detail, as are matters relating to the use of attorneys and payment of attorneys' fees. Placement of the child during pendency of the dispute is also discussed.

I. MEDIATION

The 1997 Amendments to the IDEA require Local Education Agencies to ensure that procedures are established and implemented to allow disputes relating to the evaluation, placement, or education of a child with a disability to be resolved through mediation whenever a due process hearing is requested by either party. (See part II of this chapter for an explanation of due process hearings.)

Question: **What is mediation?**

Answer: Mediation is a process whereby the parents and the school district attempt to resolve any dispute relating to the evaluation, placement, or education of a child who is deaf or hard-of-hearing, prior to undergoing formal administrative or legal action to resolve that dispute.

Question: **Must parents agree to mediate a dispute prior to seeking administrative or court relief?**

Answer: No. Mediation is voluntary on the part of the parents. And it may not be used to deny or delay parents the right to a due process hearing.

Question: **If the parties agree to mediate, how is the mediation session conducted?**

Answer: A qualified and impartial mediator trained in effective mediation techniques will conduct the mediation session. The mediator will assist parents and the school district in engaging in a meaningful discussion among themselves relating to the dispute. The mediator simply facilitates the discussion; the mediator does not make any decisions during the discussion.

Question: **Who selects the mediator?**

Answer: The state is required to maintain a list of qualified and impartial mediators to serve in IDEA disputes. In the event a mediator is needed, he or she will be selected on a random basis from that list. Both parents and school district must agree to the selection of the mediator.

Question: **If parents do not want to meet with a state mediator, what happens?**

Answer: A state or a school district *may* (but is not required to) establish procedures to require parents who choose not to use the mediation process to meet with a disinterested party who is under contract with either (a) a parent training and information center; or (b) a community parent resource center; or (c) an appropriate alternative dispute resolution entity, to explain the benefits of the mediation process to the parents and encourage the parents to use the mediation process. It remains to be seen whether all states or school districts will implement such requirements.

Question: **Can parents still decline to mediate after meeting with a required disinterested party who has explained the mediation process?**

Answer: Yes. Parents may not be compelled to submit to mediation prior to engaging in a due process hearing. In most cases, however, it would be to the parents' advantage to do so. Mediation is advisable whenever possible.

Question: **Can parents bring an attorney or advocate to the mediation process?**

Answer: The 1997 Amendments leave it up to the individual states to determine whether attorneys (and presumably advocates) may attend the mediation process. It remains to be seen what the states will do in this regard.

Question: **Who pays for the mediation process?**

Answer: The state bears the entire cost.

Question: **If the mediation process is completed, how are the results indicated?**

Answer: The agreement reached between the parties in the mediation process will be set forth in a written mediation agreement.

Question: **Is the mediation process, and all discussions that occur during that process, kept confidential?**

Answer: Yes, and that information may not be used in any later due process hearing or court proceeding. The parties to the mediation process may be required to sign a confidentiality pledge before the mediation process begins.

II. DUE PROCESS HEARINGS

Question: **What happens when parents disagree with the school district about the evaluation(s) performed of their deaf or hard-of-hearing child, the proposed placement for their child, or the provision of a free appropriate public education (FAPE) for their child, and mediation does not resolve the problem?**

Answer: When parents and school district disagree concerning the identification, evaluation, placement, or provision of a FAPE for a child with a disability (or a suspected disability), and negotiation and mediation prove unsuccessful, either may initiate a due process hearing. While later either party (the losing party in the due process hearing) may file a lawsuit against the other in state or federal court, generally—with a few exceptions—a lawsuit may not be filed until the administrative procedures (i.e., the due process hearings) have been completed.

Question: **Who conducts the due process hearing?**

Answer: The due process hearing will be conducted by the state education agency (SEA) or the local education agency (LEA), depending on state law. Some states have a two-tier administrative procedure, while other states have only a one-tier administrative procedure. In states following a two-tier procedure, the due process hearing will be held at the local level, by the LEA. The losing party may appeal the decision at a second level administrative review hearing held by the SEA. Only after there has been a decision on the matter in both administrative hearings may the losing party file an action in court. In states following a one-tier procedure the initial due process hearing is held by the SEA, and the losing party may appeal directly to the court.

The hearing must be conducted by an impartial hearing officer. To be impartial, the hearing officer may not be employed by the public agency involved in educating the child. Thus, no person employed by the SEA may be a hearing officer (regardless of whether the hearing is conducted by the SEA or the LEA). The hearing officer also may not have any other conflict of interest with respect to the hearing. Thus, for example, it has been held that a principal of a private entity that contracts with the SEA to provide services could not serve as a hearing officer due to an apparent conflict of interest.

Question: **Are hearing officers really completely impartial?**

Answer: Many commentators question whether hearing officers appointed to hear disputes arising under the IDEA are completely impartial. In some states, for example, the state department of education is solely responsible for choosing the hearing officer who will decide each individual case, and the department pays the hearing officer's fees. In those states parents are not permitted to have any input into the selection of the hearing officer. Some hearing officers, wishing to be rehired by the department of education in future cases, may be inclined to view the school district's position more kindly than the parents' position. In other situations, hearing officers are themselves educators, or are involved in the educational field in some fashion (although they do not work for the state education agency), and may have an inherent bias in favor of the positions espoused by educators.

Question: **Is there a time limit with respect to the date on which parents must request a due process hearing to challenge a school district's proposed IEP?**

Answer: No. Neither the IDEA nor the Department of Education's (DOE's) regulations establish a time frame within which parents must request a due process hearing to challenge a school district's proposed IEP. Thus parents may do so at any time.

Question: **What happens during the due process hearing?**

Answer: The due process hearing is like a mini-trial, although a little more informal than a court trial. Both the school district and the parents have the right to have an attorney present and have the right to present evidence, to bring on witnesses (and to compel the attendance of witnesses via a subpoena), and to cross examine witnesses for the other side. Evidence to be presented at the hearing must be disclosed to the other side at least 5 days before the hearing (although the hearing officer has discretion to modify the 5-day rule). If the parents requested the hearing, the parents will present their witnesses and evidence first, and the school district will follow with its evidence and witnesses. Parties can also present opening and closing arguments.

Question: **Will the due process hearing be open to the public?**

Answer: If the parents wish, they may ask that a due process hearing be open to the public. A school district may not open a due process hearing to the public if that is not in accord with the parents' wishes.

Question: **Should parents hire an attorney to represent them at the due process hearing?**

Answer: If at all possible parents should be represented by an attorney at the due process hearing. The school district will surely be represented by an attorney. Thus, parents who are not represented by an attorney will be at a severe disadvantage. Parents who are unable to afford an attorney may, in some cases, be lucky enough to find an attorney to take the case on a "contingency fee" arrangement, pursuant to which the attorney agrees not to bill the parents if they lose the case, but only to seek attorneys' fees if the parents ultimately win the case (in which case attorneys' fees will be paid for by the school district, as explained below). In many cases that will not be possible, however.

In some cases parents unable to afford or find an attorney may seek the help of a public advocate, as explained in chapter 2 of this text. An advocate is not an attorney, however, and thus if at all possible parents should secure legal representation.

Question: **If parents succeed in obtaining much of the relief sought during the due process hearing, may the school district be required to pay for the services of the parents' attorney?**

Answer: The IDEA provides that a court may, in its discretion, award reasonable attorneys' fees (as part of the costs to be paid by the school district) to the parents or guardian of a child with a disability when the parents or guardian are the successful party in the action. Thus, parents who ultimately succeed in obtaining the basic relief sought may be reimbursed by the school district for legal expenses (including attorneys' fees) incurred during any due process hearings. It is important to understand, however, that parents must be the *final* "winning" parties. Thus, if parents "win" the case at the due process hearing level, but the school district appeals to a court and ultimately the school district "wins" in court, parents will not be entitled to reimbursement for attorneys' fees incurred during the successful due process hearing. (The ruling of the *last* court to hear the case will apply.) The same rule will apply if, in a state applying a two-tier administrative process, parents "win" at the first level due process hearing but ultimately lose at the second due process hearing (or later lose in court).

Only a court can order a school district to pay the parents' attorneys' fees, however; the hearing officer cannot make such an order. Thus, parents who succeed at the administrative due process hearing level will have to file an action in court requesting that the court enter an order requiring the school district to pay the parents' attorneys' fees incurred during the administrative proceedings.

Question: **Can the school district ever be required to pay the parents attorneys' fees incurred at a due process hearing when the parents lose at the hearing?**

Answer: If parents lose at the due process hearing level and appeal their case to court and ultimately win the case in court, the school district can be compelled to reimburse parents for attorneys' fees incurred at the due process hearing, despite the fact that the parents lost in the due process hearing. Whenever parents are the final "winners" in the case they may be reimbursed for attorneys' fees incurred both at the due process hearing level and in court.

Question: **If courts have "discretion" as to whether or not to award attorneys' fees to prevailing parents (parents who won their case), might a court decide not to make the school district pay such attorneys' fees if the court feels that the school district was acting in good faith?**

Answer: The courts have held that "good faith" on the part of a school district does not take away the rights of "winning" parents to obtain attorneys' fees under the IDEA. Generally, courts award attorneys' fees to parents as a matter of routine.

Question: **If the school district ultimately wins the case, can parents be compelled to pay the school district's attorneys' fees?**

Answer: No. Parents cannot be required to pay the school district's legal costs.

Question: **What does it mean to say that parents may recover legal fees if they are ultimately the "prevailing" (i.e., the "winning") party?**

Answer: For parents to be considered prevailing parties in an action under the IDEA it is sufficient that the parents succeeded on any significant issue that achieved some of the benefits sought. Parents do not have to obtain all of the relief requested, just some significant relief.

In one case, for example, parents who wanted their child's educational placement changed from a residential school to a day school (the child had a disability other than deafness) did not succeed in obtaining that relief, but the parents did succeed in having their child's educational program revamped. That was held sufficient to make the parents prevailing parties. Parents who have succeeded in obtaining additional services for their children have been declared prevailing parties despite the fact that they did not obtain all the services they requested (such as requesting speech therapy three times a week but only obtaining such therapy two times a week).

Question: **When and how must a hearing officer announce his or her ruling after a due process hearing is completed?**

Answer: The hearing officer must reach a final decision within 45 days after a request for a hearing is received. (The parties may always agree, however, to extend that time period.) The hearing officer's decision must be in writing, and must contain findings of fact as well as conclusions of law.

Question: **If the hearing officer rules in favor of the parents, how soon must the school district implement the findings of the hearing officer (or file an appeal in court)?**

Answer: The IDEA does not specify a time by which a school district must implement a due process hearing decision or file an appeal. If the school district is not going to appeal it must implement the hearing decision as soon as possible, but in any event within a reasonable period of time. State law may specify the time during which a school district must appeal the hearing officer's decision. If that period is reasonable (such as a couple of weeks), the state rules could probably permit the school district to delay implementing the decision until after the time to appeal has expired.

Question: **If the school district does not implement the hearing officer's decision within a reasonable time, what can parents do?**

Answer: Parents would have to file an action in court to have the court order the school district to implement the hearing officer's decision.

Question: **What happens to the child while due process hearings are being conducted?**

Answer: If the dispute involves the child's placement in school, under the IDEA the "stay put" rule applies. That is, the child is to remain in his or her current placement pending resolution of the dispute. This rule is intended to prevent a "yo-yo" effect, pursuant to which the child would be yanked back and forth between placements while parents and school districts argued their respective positions in due process hearings and later in court.

Despite the stay put rule, however, parents and school district may always agree to change the child's placement while they proceed with their dispute (without prejudice to either party's position). Moreover, parents are free to remove their child from the public school program and place the child in a private school or other alternative placement at their own expense (and to seek reimbursement if appropriate, as explained in chapter 9 of this text). The stay put provision only prohibits the school district from unilaterally changing the child's placement.

In some exceptional cases, a court may rule that the stay put provision should not apply, because: (a) to leave the child in his or her current placement would cause the child irreparable injury and (b) the school district is likely to succeed on its claim that the current placement is not appropriate.

If the child is to remain in public school, the "current placement" is the placement in effect when the request for a due process hearing was filed. If the child is not yet in school, but the dispute involves the child's initial school placement, the law is unclear as to what should be considered the child's "current placement." It can be argued that the law requires that the child, with the consent of the parents, should be placed in the regular public school program until completion of all proceedings. The parents and school district may, of course, agree on an interim placement for the child.

The stay put rule, however, only applies when the child's *placement* is in dispute. If it is simply a minor change in *program* that is in dispute, rather than a change in *placement*, the stay put rule does not apply. What must be maintained is the general nature of the child's placement, not each and every element of that placement. A change in the location of the child's program—without corresponding program changes, for example—

is not generally viewed as a change in placement. But a change that will significantly affect the services or programs the child receives will be held to be a change in placement, that cannot be made until after the dispute is resolved. For example, if a school district proposed taking away all speech and auditory training for a deaf child, or if a school district proposed eliminating a sign language interpreter for a deaf child, these would probably constitute sufficiently significant changes to trigger the stay put rule.

Question: **May a school district avoid the stay put rule by simply eliminating the program that a deaf or hard-of-hearing child attends?**

Answer: The school district cannot do through the back door what it is prohibited from doing through the front door. Thus, withdrawal of funding has been held impermissible during pendency of a dispute, since even though the funding withdrawal does not constitute a direct change in placement it does *result* in a change of placement. In one very early court decision, however, the court ruled that a school could discontinue a program for purely budgetary reasons without violating the stay put rule.

Question: **If a school district places a child in a program temporarily, can that constitute a change of placement triggering the stay put provision?**

Answer: When a temporary change of placement results in a change for a period of longer than 1 month it has been considered a change in placement and thus a violation of the stay put rule. Similarly, as discussed in chapter 2 of this text, a suspension from school of more than 10 days is considered to be a change of placement triggering the stay put rule.

Question: **When a child is moving from one school district to another, and the dispute involves the child's placement**

in the new school district, what constitutes the "current placement"?

Answer: According to the Department of Education (DOE), when a child with a disability moves from one school district to another in the same state, the new school placement is not to be considered a "new admission." Thus, in that situation, the "current placement" that must be maintained is the IEP developed at the former school. At least one court has held that this same rule applies when a child moves to a new school district in another state.

Question: **What can parents do if the child's new school district will not follow the IEP established by the child's old school district?**

Answer: Parents do not have to request a due process hearing. Rather, parents can go immediately to court and ask the court to grant a preliminary injunction ordering the new school district to implement the prior IEP pending resolution of the dispute between the parents and the new school district regarding the child's placement.

III. COURT ACTIONS

Question: **If parents lose at the administrative due process hearing level, what can they do?**

Answer: Parents can file an action in state or federal court. As previously noted, however, parents generally cannot file a court action until they have first "exhausted their administrative remedies," which means that they must first have requested, and obtained, a due process hearing. In states having a two-tier administrative procedure, before parents can file a court action they must have completed two due process hearings, one before the local education agency (LEA) and another before the state education agency (SEA).

Question: **Is there a time frame during which parents must file a court action?**

Answer: The time frame during which parties must file an action in court is known as the "statute of limitations." The IDEA does not specify a statute of limitations during which actions must be filed under the Act. Thus, courts apply the state statute of limitations that applies in actions that most closely resemble actions filed under the IDEA. Depending upon the state, the statute of limitations can be anywhere from 30 days to 4 years from the date on which the "injury" occurred (the date on which the final hearing officer's decision was rendered). Parents will have to determine what the applicable statute of limitations is in their state.

Question: **If parents or the school district appeal to a court, will the case be heard and decided by a jury or a judge?**

Answer: Cases arising under the IDEA are generally heard and decided by a judge, not a jury.

Question: **What issues and evidence will the court consider on appeal?**

Answer: Courts will usually consider only those issues that were raised during the due process hearing(s) (i.e., the administrative hearing[s]). A court will not consider issues that could have been but were not raised at the administrative hearings.

With respect to what evidence will be reviewed when deciding the issues discussed at the administrative hearings, however, the courts do not always agree. Some courts will only review evidence that was presented at the administrative hearing(s), plus any directly supplemental evidence. Most courts, however, will review any new evidence that is relevant and necessary to the case (as long as the evidence deals with the same issues that were raised at the administrative hearing[s]).

Question: **Does the stay put rule apply during court proceedings as well?**

Answer: Generally, yes. The stay put rule always applies during initial court proceedings, that is, while the case is being resolved by a federal district court or a state superior court. There is some question as to whether the stay put rule applies if the party who loses the case at that court level appeals the case to a higher court (a court of appeals).

Question: **Can parents obtain attorneys' fees if they are the prevailing party in the court action?**

Answer: Yes. See the discussion about attorneys' fees in the preceding section dealing with due process hearings.

Question: **Are there limits to the amount of attorneys' fees that may be awarded?**

Answer: Yes. Attorneys' fees must be based on the prevailing rates received by other attorneys in the community who provide the same kind and quality of services. The 1997 Amendments to the IDEA provide that attorneys are not entitled to "bonuses" or "multipliers" of fees (which are sometimes awarded in certain cases for very difficult or unique cases).

Question: **If parents refuse to settle their case with the school district, can they still recover attorneys' fees?**

Answer: The 1997 Amendments provide as follows: If the school district offers in writing to settle the case 10 days before due process hearings or court proceedings begin, and the parents do not accept that offer within 10 days, and if the relief obtained by the parents is not more favorable to the parents than the settlement offer, the parents may not be awarded attorneys' fees. If, however, the hearing officer or court finds that parents who were the prevailing party were "substantially justified" in rejecting the settlement offer, the parents may recover attorneys' fees. Whether the parents were "substantially justified" in rejecting the settlement offer will be up to the hearing officer or court to decide.

Question: **Can attorneys' fees to be awarded to parents be reduced for any reason?**

Answer: Yes. Under the 1997 Amendments, the attorneys' fees to be awarded to parents may be reduced by the court if the court finds that: (a) The parents *unreasonably* prolonged resolution of the dispute; (b) the amount of attorneys' fees to be awarded are excessive in light of the time spent and the services furnished; or (c) the parents' attorney did not provide the school district with required information. Attorneys' fees will not be reduced, however, if the school district unreasonably prolonged resolution of the dispute.

CHAPTER 9

Remedies

This chapter addresses the remedies that may be obtained in the event that parents and school district officials engage in dispute resolution to resolve differences of opinion.

Question: **If parents succeed on their claims after bringing an action in court, can the parents obtain damages from the school district?**

Answer: The IDEA provides that courts "shall grant all appropriate relief." Despite this broad language, the courts are not in agreement with respect to the question of whether monetary damages are available under the Act. Some courts have held that monetary damages are available under the IDEA, while many others have held that they are not. To date, therefore, the question remains unresolved. The most recent cases, however, seem to follow the reasoning that damages are available. In addition, parents may be able to obtain damages under other laws protecting children with disabilities, such as Section 504 of the Rehabilitation Act discussed in chapter 1 of this text.

Question: **Aside from the issue of monetary damages, what remedies are available under the IDEA to parents who succeed in a legal action?**

Answer: Several remedies are available to parents who successfully pursue a legal action under the IDEA, including the following:

1. Injunctive relief is always available. That is, a hearing officer or a court may enter an order requiring the school district to implement the necessary program, provide the necessary services, or do whatever else is required to comply with the ruling.

2. Reimbursement is available for expenses incurred when parents place their child in a program that is ultimately determined to be the appropriate placement for the child. Such expenses may, in appropriate cases, include tuition costs, costs of residential placement, expenses for related services, expenses for other services necessary to allow the child to receive a FAPE (such as private tutoring), earnings or wages that a parent lost due to time spent to protect his or her child's rights, and interest on money borrowed to pay for the child's tuition or other expenses.

The United States Supreme Court has ruled that reimbursement is available even if the parents unilaterally placed their child in a private school that is not approved by the state department of education (the SEA) [Florence County School District Four v. Carter, 114 S. Ct. 361 (1993)]. When the school's proposed placement is found to be inappropriate for the child, and the parent's unilateral placement is held to be appropriate, the parents are entitled to reimbursement [Burlington School Committee of the Town of Burlington v. Department of Education of Massachusetts, 471 U.S. 359 (1985)].

Reimbursement is not considered to be a form of damages. Moreover, either a hearing officer or a court may award reimbursement.

3. Compensatory education services may be available in some circumstances. Compensatory education services are meant to remedy the progress lost by a student with a disability because he or she was previously denied a FAPE. If a student was not provided with an appropriate education for several years, for example, and as a result it is necessary for the student to attend school beyond the age at which state funded education services usually are provided, the school district may be required to provide the necessary education services to allow the student to "catch up" despite the fact that the student is "over age."

The majority of courts have held that compensatory education services are available under the IDEA. One rationale for awarding compensatory education services is that, if such a remedy is not available, parents who could not afford to unilaterally place their child in a private school (pending reimbursement in the event their claim is found to be successful) would be deprived of rights otherwise available under the IDEA. A few courts have disagreed. In those instances when a court rules that compensatory education services are not an available remedy under the IDEA, however, that remedy should be available under Section 504 of the Rehabilitation Act.

Hearing officers, as well as courts, have awarded compensatory education services.

4. Attorneys' fees are available to parents who obtain the significant relief in the action, as explained in chapter 8 of this text. As previously noted, however, only a court may award attorneys' fees; a hearing officer cannot award such fees (although the court may award attorneys' fees incurred during the due process hearings).

5. Costs incurred in resolving the dispute are also available to prevailing parents. In addition to usual costs (such as any filing or copying fees), such costs include reasonable fees and expenses of expert witnesses who come to testify on behalf of the parents' position, as well as reasonable costs for tests or evaluations of the child which are necessary to prepare the parents' case.

CHAPTER 10

Infants and Toddlers

This chapter discusses that section of the IDEA generally known as Part H, which the 1997 Amendments of the IDEA have re-labeled Part C. Part C of the IDEA (formerly Part H) governs the provision of services for deaf and hard-of-hearing infants and toddlers (from birth to age 3). Part C (formerly Part H) differs in numerous respects from Part B of the IDEA, which was discussed in the previous chapters, and which governs the provision of appropriate educational services for children age 3 or over. Accordingly, this chapter addresses the manner in which services are provided under Part C (formerly Part H), and the rights and obligations of both states and parents (on behalf of their children) under Part C (formerly Part H). Henceforth this Part will be referred to as "Part C."

Question: Part B of the IDEA only covers children who have reached the age of three. What protection does the IDEA provide for infants and toddlers, ages zero to three, who are deaf or hard-of-hearing?

Answer: Part C of the IDEA, which was established in 1986 as Part H and amended as Part C in 1997, covers children with disabilities from birth until the age of 3. States that choose to participate under Part C (to obtain federal financial assistance for infant and toddler programs) must enact a statewide system of coordinated and comprehensive programs to provide appropriate early intervention services to certain infants and toddlers with disabilities.

Question: **Who is eligible for services under Part C?**

Answer: Infants and toddlers may be eligible for Part C early intervention services or programs if they have developmental delays, are at risk of developmental delays, or have a diagnosed physical or mental condition which may result in developmental delays. Because infants and toddlers who are deaf or hard-of-hearing often suffer language delays, which may lead to further developmental delays, they are usually eligible for services under Part C.

Question: **What are the purposes of Part C?**

Answer: Part C is intended to encourage states to provide early intervention services to infants and toddlers with disabilities. The purposes of early intervention services provided under Part C are to enhance the development and adaptability of infants and toddlers with disabilities, to assist such infants and toddlers to maximize their ultimate potential, to help families meet the special needs of such infants and toddlers, and, in the long run, to reduce overall educational and developmental costs for these children.

Question: **What are the primary differences between Parts B and C of the IDEA?**

Answer: Part C, unlike Part B, is implemented and coordinated through a designated state agency which becomes the centralized agency through which all early education services are controlled. Additionally, Part C services are designed around a family-oriented plan, known as the Individualized Family Service

Plan (ISFP), rather than being designed around an individualized educational plan (the IEP) under Part B, which focuses on the individual child rather than on the child and his or her family.

Question: **Which state agency is responsible for implementing and enforcing Part C?**

Answer: It is up to each individual state to assign a particular agency responsibility for Part C. In some states the Department of Economic Security is responsible for Part C; in other states it may be the Department of Education or the Department of Social Services or some other department. Parents should contact the Governor's office to determine which agency in their state is responsible for Part C.

Question: **What "early intervention" services are to be provided under Part C?**

Answer: Early intervention services that must be provided include those that are designed to meet the individual child's needs with respect to physical development, intellectual development, language and speech development, social or emotional development and/or the development of self-help skills. These services may include, depending upon the state's specific program:

1. family training, counseling, and home visits;
2. special instruction;
3. speech-language pathology and audiology services;
4. psychological services;
5. occupational and/or physical therapy;
6. service coordination services;
7. early identification, screening, and assessment services;
8. social work services;
9. assistive technology devices and accompanying services;
10. transportation and related services necessary to enable the child or the child's family to receive early intervention services;

11. health services necessary to allow the infant or toddler to benefit from other early intervention services;
12. vision services.

This list is not exhaustive, and other services and costs related to the provision of early intervention services may also be available under a state's Part C program.

Question: **Who determines whether a particular child is eligible for Part C services?**

Answer: Eligibility for Part C services is determined by the state agency implementing programs under Part C.

Question: **How does the state agency make that determination?**

Answer: Eligibility for Part C services is based on the agency's individualized evaluation and assessment of the child's needs.

Question: **How can parents learn about Part C services available in their state?**

Answer: Each state receiving federal funding under Part C of the IDEA is required to develop a centralized directory of information outlining all early intervention services available within the state and listing all organizations or programs providing assistance to children and families available for Part C programs. The directory must be in simple, plain terms and language and must provide addresses and telephone numbers of all organizations or programs listed to allow easy access by parents or other referral sources. Parents can call the office of the Governor in their state to ask where to obtain the directory.

Question: **Who initiates the referral process for an infant or toddler to receive Part C services? May parents initiate the process?**

Answer: Infants and toddlers thought to be eligible for services under Part C may be referred to the state agency responsible for implementing Part C by any number of persons or organizations, including the parents. Hospitals, doctors, other health care providers, day care facilities, social service providers, or the parents themselves can contact the Part C agency and request that a child be evaluated and assessed for Part C services.

In addition, each state receiving federal funds under Part C must establish a child-find network and work with state and public agencies, as well as the referral providers listed above, to seek out all infants and toddlers with disabilities eligible for Part C early intervention services. As part of its child-find system, the state must implement a campaign to promote public awareness of available early intervention services.

Question: **How does the Part C process work?**

Answer: After a child has been identified as possibly eligible for Part C services and referred to the state's Part C agency (either by the parents or another agency or individual), the state agency must, within 45 days, evaluate the child for eligibility under Part C and assess what services are required for the child. The evaluation and assessment must be performed by trained clinical personnel, who are to consider the child's medical history, level of development, and the resources and concerns of the child's family.

Question: **May parents decline to participate in the evaluation process?**

Answer: Yes.

Question: May the state evaluate a child with a suspected hearing loss without the consent of the parents?

Answer: Parents must consent in writing, after being fully informed of all relevant information, to have their child evaluated. If a parent refuses to consent to the initial evaluation, the state agency may initiate a due process hearing to override the parental refusal.

Question: May parents bring their own "experts" or advocates into the evaluation and assessment process?

Answer: Neither Part C nor the federal regulations outlining the responsibilities under Part C contain a provision giving parents the right to bring outside experts or advocates into the initial evaluation and assessment process to determine whether a child is eligible for Part C services. But parents always have the right to have any complaints or disputes regarding the evaluation and assessment process heard at an impartial administrative proceeding. During any administrative proceeding the parents may retain counsel and present expert testimony or other evidence to prove their case. The administrative hearing process is discussed at the end of this chapter.

Question: What happens if the child is found eligible to receive Part C services?

Answer: If the child is found to be eligible for Part C services, within the initial 45-day period the state agency must hold a meeting with the child's family to develop an Individualized Family Service Plan (IFSP). The IFSP meeting is usually held after the initial evaluation and assessment of the child. A service coordinator will be assigned to the family.

Question: **What role does the service coordinator play?**

Answer: The state agency responsible for implementing Part C will assign a service coordinator to the family. The service coordinator is responsible for coordinating all services for the child and will serve as the person for parents to contact when seeking to obtain necessary services and assistance. The service coordinator is also required to assist parents in identifying and locating available services and service providers, and to inform parents (and families) of the availability of advocacy services.

Question: **Who participates in the IFSP meeting?**

Answer: On behalf of the state, the following people are to attend the IFSP meeting: The Part C service coordinator (sometimes called a Case Manager) (if appointed), the personnel who conducted the initial evaluation and assessment of the child and his or her family, and any known service providers who will work with the child.

The parents are expected attendees at the IFSP meeting, as well as any other family members whom the parents wish to have attend and participate. In addition, the parents may request that an advocate or other person outside the family be allowed to attend and participate.

Question: **What happens if parents wish an advocate or other person outside the family to attend the IFSP meeting, but that person is not able to attend on the scheduled date of the meeting?**

Answer: If the parents have requested an advocate or other person outside the family to attend the IFSP meeting, the meeting cannot be conducted without that person's presence. Presence may be physical, or indirect through means such as a telephone conference call or the sending of a personal representative.

Question: **What is to be contained in the IFSP?**

Answer: As previously noted, the focus of the IFSP, unlike the focus of an IEP for a child age 3 or more, is on the *family* rather than on the individual child. To satisfy this objective, the IFSP is required to contain the following:

1. Information about the child's present levels of development;
2. Information about the family's resources, priorities, and concerns;
3. The goals to be achieved for the child;
4. Criteria for evaluating the child's progress;
5. The specific early intervention services required to meet the needs of the child and his or her family;
6. The place(s) at which the early intervention services will be provided;
7. The date on which the early intervention services are to begin;
8. The anticipated duration of the early intervention services;
9. The service coordinator's name; and
10. The steps that will be taken to assist the child in making the transition from Part C to Part B (discussed later in this chapter).

Generally, the IFSP sets forth the specific services and programs to be utilized by the child and the child's family and establishes goals for development in key areas.

Question: **What role do the child's parents play in this process**?

Answer: The child's parents and the state agency responsible for implementing Part C participate equally in this process. Parents are participants at every stage of the process—during the evaluation and assessment, when developing the IFSP, and when reviewing and revising the IFSP. Parental consent is required for approval and implementation of the IFSP. Unlike under Part B, parents have the final say with respect to implementation of an IFSP under Part C.

Question: May parents refuse to accept Part C services?

Answer: Yes. Parents do not have to accept services for their children under Part C. Further, the state agency may not attempt to override the parental refusal to accept such services. Thus, although parents may be compelled to have their child evaluated, they may not be compelled to accept early intervention services for their child.

Question: How often is the IFSP reviewed, revised, or rewritten?

Answer: The IFSP is required to be reviewed every 6 months to determine whether modifications or additions should be made to the Plan, and to measure progress toward the development of established goals. It is not required that meetings be held every 6 months between parents and the state agency, however.

Rather, Part C requires that yearly meetings be held between the parents and the state agency to review the IFSP and make any necessary modifications or changes. The same rules apply to subsequent IFSP meetings that apply to the initial IFSP meeting, as discussed earlier.

Question: May parents request additional reviews of the IFSP?

Answer: Yes. Parents may request review of the IFSP at any time, regardless of the mandated biannual review periods.

Question: **If a child and his or her family require immediate early intervention services under Part C prior to the implementation of the IFSP, may such services be provided?**

Answer: Yes. A provisional IFSP may be implemented during the initial 45-day period after the child is identified as being potentially eligible for Part C services and referred to the state agency. This provisional IFSP may be implemented even before the assessment and evaluation of the child is performed (or during that assessment and evaluation period) if it is obvious that immediate services are required.

Question: **Must parents pay for early intervention services to be provided under Part C?**

Answer: Under the IDEA, the federal or state government may provide for a system of payments by families for Part C services, including a schedule of sliding fees based on income. Thus, state law will have to be examined. Even if a state has enacted a payment scheme, however, a child may not be denied services due to the family's inability to pay. Further, parents may not be charged for evaluations or assessments or for case management services.

Question: **Where are early intervention services to be provided?**

Answer: To the maximum extent appropriate, early intervention services are to be provided in "natural environments" including the child's home and community settings in which children without disabilities participate.

Question: **What is the continuing relationship, if any, between Parts B and C of the IDEA?**

Answer: A deaf or hard-of-hearing child who requires special education services is entitled to receive such services under Part B as of the date of his or her third birthday. When a child receives services under Part C prior to his or her third birthday, states are required to ensure a smooth transition to an IEP under Part B. If the parents approve, therefore, at least 90 days before the child's third birthday a meeting should be conducted between the LEA, the child's family, and the Part C lead agency to discuss a transition plan for the child. State policy can allow the IFSP to continue in effect past the child's birthday until such time as a smooth transition is made to an IEP under Part B, as long as the IFSP is consistent with the requirements for an IEP. (State law would have to be checked on this point.)

Question: **What happens if parents disagree with the state agency responsible for Part C with respect to the identification, evaluation, or placement of their infant or toddler, or if parents disagree with the state agency's determination of what constitutes appropriate early intervention services for the child or his or her family?**

Answer: That depends on state law. States can choose two methods of dispute resolution under Part C. Under the first method, the due process procedures that apply under Part B of the IDEA (explained in chapters 2 and 8) also apply under Part C. Alternatively, states may establish procedures that meet the requirements set forth in the Part H regulations developed by the Department of Education, which are similar, but not identical, to the Part B procedures.

There are four differences between the Part B and Part C regulatory procedures: (a) Under the Part C procedures the hearing officer must reach a decision within 30 days rather than 45 days; (b) under the Part C procedures states cannot have a two-tier administrative system as they can under Part B; (c) under the Part C procedures parents do not have the right to an Independent educational evaluation (IEE); and (d) under the Part C procedures parents are not entitled to recover attorneys' fees unless their child is also eligible for services under Part B.

Question: **Must records and information relating to the child be kept confidential under Part C as they must under Part B?**

Answer: Yes. Confidentiality is required under Part C as well as under Part B.

Question: **Does the stay put rule apply under Part C?**

Answer: Yes. The stay put rule under Part C is basically the same as under Part B, as explained in chapter 2 of this text. If a child has not yet received any services when the dispute arises, the child must receive only those services that are not in dispute pending resolution of the disagreement.

G L O S S A R Y

Glossary of Non-IDEA Terms

American Sign Language (ASL): A visual, spatial signed language having its own unique grammar, structure, and vocabulary.

Assistive Listening Device (ALD): A special piece of equipment that amplifies or directs sound. Such devices are usually used in combination with a person's hearing aid(s) or cochlear implant, but can also be utilized by themselves. There are numerous types of ALDs; among the best known are infrared systems and FM systems.

Auditory Trainer: A term that refers to the use of one or more types of assistive listening devices.

Auditory-Verbal: The application and management of technology, strategies, techniques, and procedures "to enable deaf and hard-of-hearing children to listen, with the assistance of hearing aids, cochlear implants, and/or other forms of amplification, to achieve the goal of oral communication."[1] This system emphasizes hearing to teach speech and language.

[1]From *Auditory-Verbal Therapy for Parents and Professionals*, W. Estabrooks (Ed.), 1994, p. 2. Washington, DC: Alexander Graham Bell Association.

Auditory-Verbal Therapist: An individual who is trained to work with deaf or hard-of-hearing individuals using the auditory verbal approach to acquiring spoken and receptive language skills.

Cochlear Implant: An electronic prosthetic device that is surgically inserted into the inner ear to partially perform the function of the cochlea by stimulating the auditory nerve neurons. Numerous electrodes in the prosthetic device are attached via a magnet and wires to an external processor and a microphone. The external processor sends coded information to the electronic prosthesis, which is a receiver-stimulator. The receiver-stimulator converts the coded information, which is passed to the electrodes and stimulates hearing nerve fibers, providing artificial sound that bypasses the nonfunctioning portion of the ear.

Cued Speech: A system of signals utilizing hand and finger signs or cues to assist individuals who speechread in differentiating between sounds that look alike on the lips. Eight manual cues represent invisible elements of speech. The eight manual cues cannot be utilized alone in the absence of speechreading; the two must be used together.

FM System: A frequency-modulation (FM) assistive listening system or device that operates like a radio to increase a desired signal or speech over interfering background noise. The speaker wears a transmitter/microphone, and the deaf or hard-of-hearing person wears a receiver. (*See* Assistive Listening Device.)

Infrared System: A wireless system that sends a radio signal to a battery-powered receiver. It operates only in the room in which the system is installed and is primarily used in large areas, such as concert halls, auditoriums, large conference rooms and theaters. Like the FM system, the purpose is to improve the signal to noise ratio.

Integrated Education (also known as "*Inclusion*"): Placement of a child who is deaf or hard-of-hearing primarily in the regular education classroom. The deaf or hard-of-hearing child is provided with an adapted curriculum. Thus, unlike the child in a mainstreamed setting, the deaf or hard-of-hearing child in an integrated educational setting is not expected to keep pace with hearing children in the classroom or to achieve all the regular educational requisites to move to the next class. The focus is on the deaf or hard-of-hearing child's *own* abilities.

Mainstreaming: Educating children who are deaf or hard-of-hearing in the general school setting with their normally hearing peers, following the same curriculum.

Oral Communication: Spoken and receptive communication via the use of speech (without any sign language).

Oral Interpreter: An individual who sits facing a deaf or hard-of-hearing person who communicates orally and silently mouths the words of a non-speechreadable speaker. The deaf or hard-of-hearing person speechreads the words of the oral interpreter rather than of the speaker.

Resource Teacher: An individual who works with a deaf or hard-of-hearing student on a scheduled or as-needed basis to assist the student with his or her studies. The resource teacher may or may not be specially trained to work with deaf or hard-of-hearing students. This teacher will fill in the gaps that the student has missed due to his or her hearing loss, and/or will work with the student on special language or vocabulary problems involved in course work that have arisen due to the student's hearing loss. The resource teacher thus serves as a special type of tutor.

Signed English or Signing Exact English (SEE): The use of sign language following English structure, grammar, and vocabulary word-for-word as spoken in English (unlike ASL, it does not involve a unique language).

Sign-language Interpreter: An individual who sits facing a deaf or hard-of-hearing person who communicates via sign language and signs the words of a speaker who does not sign. A sign language interpreter must sign in the sign language that the deaf or hard-of-hearing individual uses (i.e.,

ASL, signed English). A sign language interpreter will "reverse interpret" for the deaf or hard-of-hearing person if he or she does not speak for him or herself. In that case, the sign language interpreter will read the signs of the deaf or hard-of-hearing person and repeat them in voice for non-signing individuals.

Total Communication: Spoken and receptive communication via all forms of communication, usually involving primarily sign language with minimal speech and speechreading.

TTY (or TDD): Teletypewriter for the deaf (TTY), or telecommunication device for the deaf (TDD). When using a TTY or TDD, the telephone receiver is placed into two headset cups (similar to a modem) on a machine that resembles a small typewriter with a video screen and/or paper printout. The TTY (TDD) user types a message on a keyboard, which is relayed to a party on the other end of the line with a similar device. The receiver returns his or her message by typing it to the sender and the conversation proceeds via typewriter and video screen or printout.

A P P E N D I X

Organizations Providing Legal Assistance or Referrals to or for People Who Are Deaf or Hard-of-Hearing

NATIONAL

Alexander Graham Bell Association for the Deaf
3417 Volta Place, NW
Washington, DC 20007
V/TTY: 202–337–5220

American Bar Association
750 N. Lakeshore Drive
Chicago, IL 60611
Voice: 312–988–5000
TTY: 312–988–5168

National Atty. Referral Service
Voice: 800–285–2221

Lead Line - House Ear Institute
(National Information and Referral)
2100 W. 3rd Street, 5th Floor
Los Angeles, CA 90057
V/TTY: 800-352-8888 (National)
V/TTY: 800-287-4763 (in California)

National Association of the Deaf Law Center
814 Thayer
Silver Springs, MD 20910
Voice: 301–587–1788
TTY: 301–587–1789

ALABAMA

University of Alabama
College of Law
Alabama Disabilities Advocacy Program
526 Martha Parham West
Tuscaloosa, AL 35487
V/TTY: 205–348–4928

ALASKA

Disability Law Center of Alaska
615 E. 82nd Avenue, #101
Anchorage, AK 99518
V/TTY: 907–344–1002
Voice: 800–478–1234 (in Alaska)

ARIZONA

Arizona Center for Disability Law
3839 N. 3rd Street, #209

Phoenix, AZ 85012
Voice: 602–274–6287

Arizona Center for Disability Law
3131 N. Country Club, #100
Tucson, AZ 85716
Voice: 520–327–9547

Arizona Council for the Hearing Impaired
1400 W. Washington, #126
Phoenix, AZ 85007
V/TTY: 602–542–3323

ARKANSAS

Arkansas Office for the Deaf and Hard-of-Hearing
5326 W. Markham, #1
Little Rock, AR 72205
V/TTY: 501–296–1894

CALIFORNIA

California Center for Law and the Deaf
14895 E. 14th Street, #220
San Leandro, CA 94578
V/TTY: 510–483–0922

Greater Los Angeles Council on Deafness (GLAD)
2222 Laverna Avenue
Los Angeles, CA 90041
V/TTY: 213–478–8000

NORCAL Center on Deafness
1820 Tribute Road, Suite A
Sacramento, CA 95815–4307
V/TTY: 916–973–8448

COLORADO

Colorado Center on Deafness
1900 Grant Street, Suite 1010
Denver, CO 80203
V/TTY: 303–839–8022

CONNECTICUT

INFOLINE Information and Referral
1344 Silas Deane Highway
Rocky Hill, CT 06067
V/TTY: 860–522–4636
V/TTY: 800–203–1234 (in Connecticut)

DELAWARE

Community Legal Aid Society, Inc.
Disability Law Program
913 Washington Street
Wilmington, DE 19801
Voice: 302–575–0660
V/TTY: 800–575–0660 (in Delaware)

DISTRICT OF COLUMBIA

Rehabilitation Services Administration
Communication Impairment Section
800 9th Street, SW, 4th Floor
Washington, DC 20024
V/TTY: 202–645–5847

FLORIDA

Advocacy Center for Persons with Disabilities
2671 Executive Center Circle, West
Suite 100
Tallahassee, FL 32301

Voice: 800–342–0823 (in Florida)
TTY: 800–346–4127 (in Florida)

GEORGIA

Georgia Council for the Hearing Impaired, Inc.
4151 Memorial Drive, #103B
Decatur, GA 30032
V/TTY: 404–292–5312
V/TTY: 800–541–0710 (in Georgia)

HAWAII

Protection and Advocacy Agency of Hawaii
1580 Makaloa Street, #1060
Honolulu, HI 96814
V/TTY: 808–949–2922
V/TTY: 800–882–1057 (in Hawaii)

ILLINOIS

CARPLS Legal Referral Hot Line
Voice: 312–738–9200
(Answered 9 a.m.–1 p.m., M–F)

IDAHO

COAD (Protection and Advocacy)
4477 Emerald, Suite B-100
Boise, ID 83706
V/TTY: 208–336–5353
V/TTY: 800–632–5125 (in Idaho)

INDIANA

Deaf and Hard-of-Hearing Services
V/TTY: 317–232–1143
V/TTY: 800–962–8408 (in Indiana)

Indiana Protection and Advocacy Services
4701 N. Keystone Ave., #22
Indianapolis, IN
Voice: 317–722–5555
Voice: 800–622–4845 (in Indiana)
TTY: 800–838–1131 (in Indiana)

IOWA

Deaf Services Commission of Iowa
Iowa Department of Human Rights
Lucas State Office Bldg.
Des Moines, IA 50319
V/TTY: 515–281–3164

KANSAS

Kansas Commission for the Deaf and Hard-of-Hearing
Biddle Bldg., 1st Floor
300 SW Oakley
Topeka, KS 66606–1861
V/TTY: 913–296–2874
V/TTY: 800–432–0698 (in Kansas)

KENTUCKY

Kentucky Commission on the Deaf and Hard-of-Hearing
632 Versailles Road
Frankfort, KY 40601
V/TTY: 502–573–2604
V/TTY: 800–256–1523 (in Kentucky)

Legal Aid Society
425 W. Muhammad Ali Blvd.
Louisville, KY 40202
Voice: 502–584–1254
TTY: 502–584–6750

LOUISIANA

Governor's Office of Disability Affairs
P. O. Box 94004
Baton Rouge, LA 70804
V/TTY: 504–342–1683

MAINE

Maine Advocacy Services
P.O. Box 2007
Augusta, ME 04338–2007
V/TTY: 207–626–2774
V/TTY: 800–452–1948 (in Maine)

MARYLAND

Maryland Disability Law Center
1800 N. Charles Street, #204
Baltimore, MD 21201
Voice: 410–234–2791

MASSACHUSETTS

Massachusetts Commission for the Deaf and Hard of Hearing
Advocacy and Legal Referrals
210 South Street, 5th Floor
Boston, MA 02111
V/TTY: 617–695–7500
TTY: 800–530–7570 (in Massachusetts)
Voice: 800–882–1155 (in Massachusetts)

MICHIGAN

Division on Deafness
320 N. Washington Square
Lansing, MI 48909
V/TTY: 517–334–7363
V/TTY: 800–729–2253 (in Michigan)

MINNESOTA

Minnesota Disability Law Center
430 First Avenue North, Suite 300
Minneapolis, MN 55401
Voice: 612–332–1141
TTY: 612–332–4668
Voice: 800–292–4150 (in Minnesota)

MISSISSIPPI

Mississippi Protection and Advocacy System, Inc.
5330 Executive Place, Suite A
Jackson, MS 39206
V/TTY: 601–981–8207
V/TTY: 800–772–4057 (in Mississippi)

MISSOURI

Commission for the Deaf
915 Leslie Blvd., Suite E
Jefferson City, MO 65101
V/TTY: 573–526–5205
V/TTY: 800–796–6499 (in Missouri)

Missouri Protection and Advocacy
925 S. Country Club Dr.
Jefferson City, MO 65109
V/TTY: 573–893–3333
V/TTY: 800–392–8667 (in Missouri)

MONTANA

Montana Advocacy Program
316 N. Park, Room 211
Helena, MT 59624
V/TTY: 406–444–3889
V/TTY: 800–245–4743 (in Montana)

NEBRASKA

Nebraska Commission for the Hearing Impaired
4600 Valley Road, #420
Lincoln, NE 68510
V/TTY: 402–471–3593
V/TTY: 800–545–6244 (in Nebraska)

NEVADA

Nevada Office of Community Based Services, Information and Referral
711 S. Stewart Street
Carson City, NV 89701
Voice: 702–687–4452
TTY: 702–687–3388
V/TTY: 888–337–3839 (in Nevada)

NEW HAMPSHIRE

Disabilities Rights Center, Inc.
Advocacy and Legal Assistance
18 Low Avenue
Concord, NH 03301
V/TTY: 603–228–0432
V/TTY: 800–834–1721 (in New Hampshire)

NEW JERSEY

Division of the Deaf and Hard of Hearing
CN #074
Trenton, NJ 08625
V/TTY: 609–984–7281
V/TTY: 800–792–8839 (in New Jersey)

NEW MEXICO

New Mexico Commission for the Deaf and Hard of Hearing,
 Information and Referral

1435 St. Francis Drive
Sante Fe, NM 87505
V/TTY: 505–827–7588
V/TTY: 800–489–8536 (in New Mexico)

NEW YORK

New York State Office of Advocate for Persons with Disabilities
One Empire State Plaza, Suite 1001
Albany, NY 12223–1150
V/TTY: 800–522–4369

NORTH CAROLINA

Department of Human Resources
Division of Services for the Deaf/HOH
319 Chapanoke Road, #108
Raleigh, NC 27603
V/TTY: 919–773–2963

NORTH DAKOTA

Office of Vocational Rehabilitation
Disability Services Division
600 S. 2nd Street, #1B
Bismarck, ND 58504
Voice: 701–328–8950
V/TTY: 701–328–8968
V/TTY: 800–755–2745 (in North Dakota)

OHIO

Ohio Legal Rights Service
8 East Long Street, 5th Floor
Columbus, OH 43215
V/TTY: 614–466–7264
V/TTY: 800–282–9181 (in Ohio)

OKLAHOMA

Oklahoma Disability Law Center, Inc.
300 Cameron Bldg.
2915 Classen Blvd.
Oklahoma City, OK 73106
V/TTY: 405–525–7755
V/TTY: 800–880–7755 (in Oklahoma)

OREGON

Oregon Disabilities Commission
1257 Ferry Street, SE
Salem, OR 97310
V/TTY: 503–378–2272
V/TTY: 800–358–3117 (in Oregon)

PENNSYLVANIA

Office for the Deaf and Hard-of-Hearing
1308 Labor and Industry Blvd.
Seventh & Forester Streets
Harrisburg, PA 17120–0019
V/TTY: 717–783–4912
V/TTY: 800–233–3008 (in Pennsylvania)

RHODE ISLAND

Protection and Advocacy System
151 Broadway
Providence, RI 02903
Voice: 401–831–3150
TTY: 401–831–5335

Commission on the Deaf and Hard-of-Hearing
One Capitol Hill, 2nd Floor
Providence, RI 02908

Voice: 401–277–1204
TTY: 401–277–1205

SOUTH CAROLINA

Protection and Advocacy for People with Disabilities, Inc.
3710 Landmark Drive, #208
Columbia, SC 29204
V/TTY: 803–782–0639
V/TTY: 800–922–5225 (in South Carolina)

SOUTH DAKOTA

Communication Services for the Deaf
102 N. Krohn Place
Sioux Falls, SD 57103
V/TTY: 605–367–5760
V/TTY: 800–642–6410 (in South Dakota)

TENNESSEE

Tennessee Protection and Advocacy Services, Inc.
P.O. Box 121257
Nashville, TN 37212
V/TTY: 615–298–1080
V/TTY: 800–342–1660 (in Tennessee)

TEXAS

Advocacy, Inc.
7800 Shoal Creek Blvd., #171E
Austin, TX 78757
Voice: 512–454–4816
TTY: 512–454–0036
V/TTY: 800–252–9108 (in Texas)

UTAH

Disability Law Center
455 East 400 South, #410

Salt Lake City, UT 84111
V/TTY: 801–363–1347
V/TTY: 800–662–9080 (in Utah)

VERMONT

Disability Law Project and Client Assistance Program
264 N. Winooski Ave.
Burlington, VT 05402
V/TTY: 802–863–2881
V/TTY: 800–252–9108 (in Texas)

VIRGINIA

Department for the Rights of Virginians with Disabilities
202 N. 9th Street, 9th Floor
Richmond, VA 23219
V/TTY: 804–225–2042
V/TTY: 800–55–3962 (in Virginia)

WASHINGTON

Office of Deaf and Hard-of-Hearing Services
P.O. Box 45300
Olympia, WA 98504-5300
V/TTY: 360–902–8000
TTY: 360–753–0699
Voice: 800–422–7930 (in Washington, Message Only)

WEST VIRGINIA

West Virginia Advocates, Inc.
1207 Quarrier Street, 4th Floor
Charleston, WV 25301–1842
V/TTY: 304–346–0847
V/TTY: 800–950–5250 (in West Virginia)

WISCONSIN

Wisconsin Coalition for Advocacy, Inc.
16 N. Carroll, Suite 400
Madison, WI 53703
V/TTY: 608–267–0214
V/TTY: 800–928–8778 (in Wisconsin)

WYOMING

Protection and Advocacy System, Inc.
2424 Pioneer Avenue, #101
Cheyenne, WY 82001
V/TTY: 307–632–3496
V/TTY: 800–624–7648